PROSTATE CANCER 20/20

A PRACTICAL GUIDE TO UNDERSTANDING MANAGEMENT OPTIONS FOR PATIENTS AND THEIR FAMILIES

ANDREW L. SIEGEL, M.D.

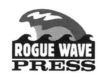

ROGUE WAVE
PRESS

Published by ROGUE WAVE PRESS

First edition 2019

ISBN: 978-0-9830617-7-9

To order additional copies of this book: www.AndrewSiegelMD.com

Cover design by Jeff Siegel. Cover image courtesy of Rost-9 / Bigstockphoto.com.

DISCLAIMER: This publication contains the opinions, ideas, and biases of the author, with the intent of providing informative materials on the topics addressed. There is no intent that any of the information provided should be construed as medical advice or professional medical services. Before adopting any recommendations made in the book, it is imperative that the reader consult with his or her own health care provider. The author and publisher disclaim any and all responsibility for any liability, loss or risk incurred as a consequence of the use of and application of any of the contents of the book.

Table of Contents

Dedication

This book is dedicated to you—the man who has been diagnosed with prostate cancer—and your partner, family and friends who support you. Strength, courage and grit are necessary to confront any cancer, most certainly when it involves such a deep-seated, mysterious and intimate organ as the prostate.

This book is also dedicated to the 3 million prostate cancer survivors in the United States and the legions of worldwide survivors who have bravely faced the daunting process of diagnosis, treatment and follow-up, a lifelong commitment. Included in this group are the prostate cancer patients for whom I provide ongoing urological care, representing about one of every five patients in my practice. These patients have been among my most important teachers and have provided me with a wealth of information not found in medical textbooks or journals, nor taught in medical school or during urology residency.

Finally, I dedicate this book to my father—Jerald Siegel—a retired urologist who is included in the ranks of prostate cancer survivors. Fortunately, more than twenty years after treatment he is alive, well and thriving, as are the vast majority of men who are treated for prostate cancer.

Acknowledgments

A heartfelt thank you to Les, my faithful partner, steadfast helpmate, collaborator, confidante, editor, tandem bike mate and best friend. She has always been an unwavering advocate who has provided me with unconditional support, never begrudging me the substantial amounts of time I have spent pursuing my passions. She has been a source of clarity, solace and sustenance and a loving and stalwart fixture in a world too often marked by randomness, chaos and lunacy. Her experience in the publishing field as an editor at Prentice Hall and director of publicity and promotion at Random House prior to becoming a mom and CEO of our household have been of great benefit in terms of converting my rambling into coherent prose and medical mumbo-jumbo into readable English. For all of this, and so much more, I am forever grateful.

I am indebted and beholden to my mentors Dr. Alan J. Wein and Dr. Shlomo Raz. Dr. Wein is co-director of the urologic oncology and voiding function and dysfunction programs and Professor of Urology at Perelman School of Medicine at the University of Pennsylvania, where I completed my urology residency. Dr. Wein instilled intellectual curiosity, a vigorous work ethic and the philosophy of aggressive diagnostic testing with conservative surgical management. To this day, when confronted with a challenging clinical situation, I silently muse to myself: what would A.J.W. do? Dr. Raz is recently retired Professor of Pelvic Medicine and Reconstruction at David Geffen School of Medicine at UCLA, where I pursued fellowship training following residency. Dr. Raz inculcated the beauty of simplicity, the importance of questioning dogma, the value of maintaining flexibility to enable constant modification and evolution, as well as the harmonious blending of the joys of living and working.

I am grateful to Dr. Louis B. Harrison, chairman of the Department of Radiation Oncology and Chief of Radiation Oncology service at Moffitt Cancer Center, who graciously wrote the foreword. He oversees all clinical and research programs at Moffitt and in 2017 was name by the American Society for Radiation Oncology (ASTRO) as a Gold Medalist, the highest honor bestowed upon ASTRO members who have made outstanding lifetime achievements in clinical patient care, research, teaching and service to the profession.

My great appreciation to Dr. Glen Gejerman, Director of Prostate Radiation Oncology at Hackensack Meridian Health–Hackensack University Medical Center who also serves as Medical Director of Radiation Oncology at New Jersey Urology, for his efforts in reviewing and editing the radiation therapy chapter. Gratitude to Dr. Robert Alter and Dr. James Orsini, medical oncologists for reviewing and editing the castration resistant prostate cancer chapter. Dr. Alter specializes in urological oncology and practices at the John Theurer Cancer Center at Hackensack Meridian Health–Hackensack University Medical Center. Dr. Orsini is a clinical oncologist with Essex Oncology who serves as the advanced prostate cancer oncologist with New Jersey Urology. A hearty thanks to Dr. Ivan Grunberger for his assistance in reviewing and editing the chapter on high intensity focused ultrasound. Dr. Grunberger is Chief of Urology at New York Presbyterian Brooklyn-Methodist Hospital and Professor of Clinical Urology at Cornell Weill Medical College and an Adjunct Professor of Urology at SUNY Downstate Medical School. Kudos to Dr. Robert Waxman, New Jersey Imaging Network radiologist and expert in multiparametric prostate MRI, for his assistance with the prostate MRI chapter. Credit to Dr. Steven Peters, Director of Anatomic Pathology at Rutgers New Jersey Medical School, for helping distill the complexity of cancer into simple and understandable terms.

Hats off to Paul Nelson—male sexual educator, advocate, coach (TheED-Coach.com), president of the Erectile Dysfunction Foundation and creator of Frank Talk (FrankTalk.org)—for his collaboration on the sexual dysfunction section. Recognition to Niva Herzig, pelvic floor physiotherapist and the director of Core Dynamics physical therapy in Englewood and Hoboken, New Jersey, for her contributions on pelvic floor physical therapy.

An ocean of thanks to my urology partners—Dr. Chris Wright, Dr. Thomas Christiano, Dr. Gregory Lovallo, Dr. Mutahar Ahmed, Dr. Michael Esposito, Dr. Martin Goldstein and Dr. Vincent Lanteri—for their assistance with the chapter on robotic-assisted laparoscopic prostatectomy and their presence as a collaborative team to provide optimal care to patients with complex urological problems.

Creative credit goes to Mohesh K. Mohan for his excellent medical illustrations. Finally, a tremendous debt of gratitude to four-time Emmy award winner Jeffrey Siegel for his assistance with all things technical including the book cover, e-book, print-on-demand book and trailer.

Common Abbreviations

ADT: androgen deprivation therapy

AS: active surveillance

ASAP: atypical small acinar proliferation

AUS: artificial urinary sphincter

BMD: bone mineral density

BMI: body mass index

BC: bulbocavernosus muscle

CRPC: castrate resistant prostate cancer

CT: computerized tomography

DNA: deoxyribonucleic acid

DRE: digital rectal exam

ED: erectile dysfunction

HDR: high dose rate brachytherapy

HGPIN: high grade prostate intraepithelial neoplasia

IGRT: image guided radiation therapy

IMRT: intensity modulated radiation therapy

IC: ischiocavernosus muscle

LHRH: luteinizing hormone-releasing hormone

LDR: low dose rate brachytherapy

LUTS: lower urinary tract symptoms

MRI: magnetic resonance imaging

NVB: neuro-vascular bundles

PET: positron emission tomography

PFM: pelvic floor muscle(s)

PSA: prostate specific antigen

PSADT: prostate specific antigen doubling time

PSMA: prostate specific membrane antigen

PTI: percent of tumor involvement

RALP: robotic-assisted laparoscopic prostatectomy

RT: radiation therapy

SRE: skeletal related events

SUI: stress urinary incontinence

VED: vacuum erection device

Foreword

The diagnosis of prostate cancer can lead to tremendous stress and confusion. After absorbing the shock of a cancer diagnosis, every man who has received this news must then decide what to do. Does my prostate cancer even require treatment? Should I have surgery or radiation? If I have radiation, what techniques should be employed? What about hormone therapy? How do I decide who to trust to take care of me?

These are big questions, and the answers to these questions will have profound consequences to the patient. Unfortunately, not every patient gets a fair chance to get honest and unbiased answers. Too many practitioners in both urology and radiation oncology are too biased about their own methods of treatment and do not present a fair analysis. Patients often seek to "break the tie" by getting more opinions or seeking advice from their primary care physician—a seemingly neutral party.

Dr. Siegel has worked hard to create a valuable resource to men who are trying to figure out the answers to these questions. In this book, he presents a fair and informative guide for men who have been diagnosed with prostate cancer… and for those who love them as well. Reading this book can be an invaluable component of making the right decision at a very difficult time.

Of note, Dr. Siegel and I share a common thread. Besides being friends for several decades, both of our fathers are long term survivors of prostate cancer. Ironically, Dr. Siegel is a urologist and I am a radiation oncologist. One of our fathers chose surgery and the other chose radiation therapy (who chose which is not relevant!). Both are alive, well and happy, many years later—testimony to good decision making. If this book was available to them decades ago, their decisions would have been much simpler.

Good luck in your journey.

Louis B. Harrison MD, FASTRO

Chair and Senior Member, Department of Radiation Oncology

Moffitt Cancer Center and Research Institute, Tampa, Florida

Preface

This book originated in the form of a 50-page monograph on prostate cancer that I crafted for my patients about a decade ago. It was conceived out of frustration from the lack of availability of a streamlined, practical, accessible and trustworthy medical resource to help patients and their families navigate through the formidable process of prostate cancer diagnosis and management. The manual proved to be beneficial for my patients and those of my urology partners and was reprinted in 2011.

With few copies remaining and time for a reprint, I recognized that since the previous iteration there have been an unprecedented number of advances in prostate cancer diagnosis and management. These include improvements in screening, increasingly sophisticated imaging techniques, the development of genomic and genetic testing, the availability of an array of new medications, continued technical advances in surgical, radiation and focal therapies and the blossoming of the era of "active surveillance."

Because of the need for a major content update, I decided to expand the monograph into a more comprehensive format that could be of value not only to the patients in my urology practice, but also to any man confronting the challenges of a prostate cancer diagnosis. I aimed to stay true to my original goals of providing a concise, straightforward and easily understandable resource.

Because most patients with prostate cancer have an excellent prognosis, the long-term consequences of the disease are often, in fact, the side effects of treatment. Therefore, I considered it vital to provide in-depth information on the most common complications following treatment, namely sexual dysfunction and urinary incontinence, quality of life issues that are often given short shrift or neglected in the patient education process. Furthermore, I elected to cover the important topic of bone health, which can be compromised by prostate cancer itself, as well as by some of the treatments for the disease.

The title of the book is the same as that of the preceding monograph, with the exception of the addition of "20/20." I did so to specify the year that looms in the near future, signifying the up-to-date content, and secondly to refer to "20/20" vision, the clarity and perspective that I wish to impart.

Along with my professional relationship with prostate cancer, I also have a personal relationship with it. In 1997, the senior partner in my urology group practice—my father—was diagnosed with prostate cancer. The news was shocking to me and I clearly remember the day of diagnosis and the long run I went on to help me process it. Fortunately, he was successfully treated with an open radical prostatectomy and today is a thriving octogenarian. Despite this, the emotional events of the day of his surgery, my interaction with his surgeon, his time in the hospital, the drive home on his day of discharge, and my removal of his surgical drain, skin staples and catheter will be forever seared into my memory.

Every case of prostate cancer is unique and has a variable biological behavior, which creates the need for treatment that is individualized and nuanced. The bewildering array of management options available can cause a great deal of confusion for the individual (and his family, friends and others who support him) grappling with trying to determine how best to be treated. My intent is to provide you with knowledge and information to help guide you through your therapeutic journey, reviewing the advantages and disadvantages of each management option in as impartial a means as is possible. Being informed empowers you to be actively involved as a participant in decisions about your care, which enables you to choose the option that is best suited for you in order to minimize decisional conflict and regret.

Be Well.

Dr. Andrew L. Siegel

Section I: Prostate Cancer

Chapter 1: What is Cancer?

Cancer is the uncontrolled and disorganized growth of abnormal cells, as opposed to the controlled and organized means of replacing old cells after they become non-functional. Whereas normal cells grow, divide and die in an orderly fashion, cancer cells continue to grow, divide and form new abnormal cells.

Normal cells become cancer cells (malignant cells) when permanent mutations in the DNA (deoxyribonucleic acid) sequence of a gene transform them into a growing and destructive version of their former selves. These abnormal cells can then divide and proliferate aberrantly and without control. Although damaged DNA can be inherited, it is much more common for DNA damage to occur by exposure to environmental toxins or from random cellular events. Under normal circumstances, the body repairs damaged DNA, but with cancer cells the damaged DNA is unable to be repaired.

As cancer cells grow they form a mass of cells (1 cubic centimeter of cancer consists of about 100 million cells) and the properties of the mutated cells allow them to encroach upon, invade and damage neighboring tissues. They can also break off from their site of origin via blood and lymphatic vessels and travel to and invade remote organs including lymph glands, liver, bone and brain, a situation known as metastasis.

Chapter 2: Shocking News: "You have prostate cancer."

One's response to hearing the four words: "You have prostate cancer" is often predictable, although every reaction is unique. The initial feelings are usually shock, disbelief, confusion, numbness and even denial. Concerns and questions immediately surface, prompted by lack of information and fear of the unknown and of what the future might hold: How can this be possible? Why me? How can this be when I have no symptoms or pain? Is this an error? Was my pathology report confused with that of another man? What is my prognosis? Can I be cured? Will I be alive to see my children married? How will treatment affect my lifestyle? Will I be able to continue functioning as a man? Will I lose urinary control? How long do I have to live? How is this going to affect my ability to work?

One of my patient's responses was noteworthy—in a rich Irish brogue: "Jesus Christ, I'm going to go back to drinking and smoking."

When a man is told he has the "C-word"—one of the most loaded words in the English language—his reflex response is often to want immediate action against such a potentially life-altering diagnosis that is capable of stealing precious time from the days he is granted on this planet. However, immediate action is neither desirable nor necessary since in most cases "time is on your side" and it is important to allow a sufficient period of time to become educated and informed about prostate cancer and to process the diagnosis and the various treatment options.

One's reaction will continue to evolve over time and most men will experience discrete emotional stages, similar to those experienced during the process of grieving. Shock is followed by anger, distress, anxiety, irritability, sadness and perhaps depression and feelings of powerlessness. During this period, it is not uncommon to feel overwhelmed, lethargic and fatigued. Many men experience difficulty concentrating, insomnia and lose interest in sex.

Ultimately, one comes to terms with and accepts the reality of the diagnosis, particularly with the realization that most men with prostate cancer will go on to live long and healthy lives with fewer side effects than in previous years because of advances in treatment. Although prostate cancer can be a deadly disease for some men, it has one of the highest survival rates of any cancer, with a 99% 5-year and a 96% 15-year survival rate.

Chapter 3: Introduction

Prostate cancer is the most common malignancy—aside from skin cancer—among men in most western populations, with an estimated 165,000 new cases in 2018 in the United States. It is the second leading cause of cancer death, with an estimated 30,000 deaths in 2018 (lung cancer is the leading cause).

Fact: In my home state of New Jersey it is estimated that in 2018 there will be 5,430 new cases of prostate cancer and 750 deaths.

To put this in perspective, heart disease claims more than 600,000 lives per year in American men and is the leading cause of death in men with prostate cancer. Even in the population of men with prostate cancer, many more men die with it than of it. In fact, there are almost 3 million prostate cancer survivors in the U.S.

The major risk factors for prostate cancer are *age, race, family history*, and *lifestyle*. The likelihood of developing prostate cancer increases with aging—the greatest risk factor for prostate cancer—thought to be due to accumulation of DNA mutations from oxidative damage (literally "rusting") of prostate cells. With each decade of aging, the occurrence of prostate cancer increases considerably. More than 60% of men are 65 years old or older at the time of diagnosis, with average age at diagnosis in the late 60s.

African American men have the highest incidence of prostate cancer,1.6 times that of Caucasian men in the U.S.; furthermore, the death rate for African American men is 2.4 times higher than that of Caucasian men. On a worldwide basis, the greatest occurrence of prostate cancer is in North America and Scandinavia and the lowest in Asia. Prostate cancer is approximately 8 times more prevalent in Western countries than it is in Eastern countries.

Prostate cancer tends to run in families, so it is vital that male children of prostate cancer patients get checked annually starting at age 40 with a PSA blood test and a digital rectal exam of the prostate. (It is my belief that all men should receive an initial baseline PSA and digital rectal exam at age 40.) Risk increases according to the number of affected family members (the more affected, the higher the risk), their degree of relatedness (brother and/ or father affected confer a higher risk than cousin and/or uncle) and the age at which they were diagnosed (relatives of patients diagnosed younger than 55 years old are at highest risk). If you have a brother or a father with prostate cancer, your risk of developing it is doubled. If you have three family members with prostate cancer, or if the disease occurs in three generations in your family, or if two of your first-degree relatives have been diagnosed at an age younger than 55 years, you have a good likelihood for having hereditary prostate cancer, which confers a 50% risk of developing the disease.

My father, a retired urologist, was diagnosed with prostate cancer at age 65 and is currently 87 years old and thriving. I have been especially diligent in seeing my internist annually for a PSA blood test and a digital rectal exam of the prostate. Additionally, I have been proactive in taking a medication—to be discussed later—to decrease my risk for prostate cancer.

An unhealthy lifestyle is an additional risk factor for prostate cancer. Being overweight or obese and consuming a Western-style diet full of calorie-laden, nutritionally-empty selections (fast food, highly processed and refined foods, excessive sugars, etc.) puts one at greater risk for aggressive prostate cancer as well as dying from prostate cancer. Asian men who reside in Asian countries have the lowest risk for prostate cancer; however, after migrating to Western countries, their risk increases substantially. This is highly suggestive that diet and other lifestyle factors play a strong role in the development of prostate cancer.

Prostate cancer is unique among tumors in that it exists in two forms: *latent* (evident on autopsy studies, but not causing an abnormal rectal exam or PSA), present in 60-70% of men older than 80; and *clinically evident* (causing an abnormal rectal exam or elevated PSA), affecting about 1 in 9 men in the U.S. Overall, men have a roughly 11% chance of being diagnosed with prostate cancer and a 3% chance of dying from it. This high ratio of prostate cancer occurrence rate to death rate suggests that many of these cancers do not threaten one's life and are "indolent" cancers.

Currently, most prostate cancers are detected by PSA screening. Widespread PSA blood testing has resulted in the increased diagnosis of early, asymptomatic prostate cancer with a reduction in the prostate cancer death rate. This is as opposed to the pre-PSA era when most cancers were detected via an abnormal prostate exam or symptoms due to advanced prostate cancer.

Screening is of vital importance because localized prostate cancer typically causes no symptoms or warning signs whatsoever. Prostate cancer is most commonly diagnosed by a biopsy prompted because of a PSA elevation, an accelerated increase in the PSA over time, or an abnormal digital rectal examination (a bump, lump, hardness, asymmetry, etc.). Those prostate cancers picked up via a PSA elevation or acceleration now account for 75% of all newly diagnosed prostate cancers.

The observed trends in PSA-driven detection of prostate cancer at earlier stages and declining death rates where screening is commonly used point to the benefits of screening. If prostate cancer is not actively sought, it is not going to be found. When prostate cancer does cause symptoms, it is generally a sign of locally advanced or advanced prostate cancer and therein lies the importance of screening. The downside of screening is over-detection of low risk prostate cancer that may never prove to be problematic but may result in unnecessary treatment with adverse consequences. The downside of not screening is the under-detection of aggressive prostate cancer, with adverse consequences from necessary treatment not being given.

The challenge for those of us who treat prostate cancer is to distinguish between clinically significant ("aggressive") and clinically insignificant ("indolent") disease and to decide the best means of treating clinically significant disease to maintain quantity and quality of life.

The good news is that when detected early, clinically significant prostate cancer is highly curable. However, such prostate cancers if left untreated have a slow, steady and predictable behavior with potential for local tumor progression and spread. Death from prostate cancer is unpleasant, often involving painful cancer spread to the spine and pelvis and not uncommonly kidney and bladder obstruction. Thus, early treatment is an important consideration for men with a life expectancy exceeding 10 years. When prostate cancer is treated, it is with the intent of avoiding the long-term consequences, i.e., that which might occur 10, 15 and 20 years down the line. Even when prostate cancer is not discovered early, although not necessarily curable, it is most often a manageable condition.

I embrace the concept of the multi-disciplinary health care team approach to prostate cancer. In addition to the urologist, the physicians who specialize in prostate cancer are the radiation oncologist and the medical oncologist. This trio may be considered the prostate cancer team and are a powerful combination in terms of their ability to educate and guide management. Each member of the team has a different expertise and skillset and contributes vitally to the decision-making and management process.

Not surprisingly, physicians have inherent biases directly related to their training. In general, the urological surgeon's bias is towards favoring surgery, the radiation oncologist's is radiation therapy and the medical oncologist's is chemotherapy. I have made great efforts to get beyond my inherent surgical bias and to give honest and appropriate advice to my patients, based upon the "big picture." I strongly believe that all physicians should practice the **FBSU** test (**F**ather, **B**rother, **S**on, **U**ncle test)—giving their patients the same advice they would give to their own family members.

The Friday, June 18, 1993 *Bergen Record* newspaper published a letter to the editor that I wrote in response to an article entitled "Hazards of waiting to treat prostate cancer." The following is a verbatim transcription:

> *"I take issue with the article, 'Prostate cancer: difficult choices' (June 5), summarizing the Journal of the American Medical Association Report, which concluded that surgery or radiation, provides minimal, if any, benefits compared with watchful waiting.*
>
> *Not all prostate cancer is the same. Cancer of the prostate can behave in an indolent fashion (very slow-growing), in which case a man will die WITH prostate cancer, but not OF prostate cancer. But prostate cancer can also be aggressive, resulting in rapid progression and death: 35,000 deaths per year in American men.*
>
> *For the most indolent of prostate cancers, intervention will rarely alter the excellent prognosis. For the most aggressive of cancers, intervention will rarely alter the poor prognosis. However, in the gray zone between these two extremes exists a substantial population for which intervention will*

literally spell the difference between life and death. If physicians could accurately predict tumor behavior and potential for progression, we could more accurately choose between surgery, radiation, or watchful waiting. Unfortunately, despite great technical strides, we do NOT currently possess such a means.

Until the means and sophistication to accurately predict the behavior of individual prostate cancer becomes available, it behooves us as urologists to offer aggressive therapy to most men with this disease; otherwise, 'watchful waiting' might translate into watch the cancer and wait for progression and death."

—*Andrew Siegel MD, River Edge, New Jersey*

The writer is a urologist and an assistant clinical professor at the University of Medicine and Dentistry of New Jersey

Wow! Twenty-five years later times have certainly changed... No longer are all prostate cancers lumped together with the thought that they are the same and are best served by surgical removal. What has not changed is the variability of prostate cancer behavior: some are so unaggressive that no cure is necessary, others are so aggressive that no treatment is curative, and many fall in between these two extremes, being moderately aggressive and curable. A major advance in the last few decades is the vast improvement in the ability to predict which prostate cancers need to be actively treated and which can be watched, a nuanced and individualized approach.

Prostate cancer can be described through an analogy using birds, rabbits and turtles in a barnyard, the animals representing prostate cancers with different degrees of aggressiveness and the barnyard representing the prostate. The aim of early detection is to not allow any of the animals to escape the barnyard and cause a cancer death. The birds can easily fly away, designating the most aggressive cancers, the ones that have often spread by the time they are detected,

11

and are often not amenable to cure. On the other hand, the turtles crawl very slowly, exemplifying non-lethal cancers that can often be managed with active surveillance. The rabbits are the intermediate group that can hop out at any time, illustrating potentially lethal cancers that would likely benefit from treatment, the kind of cancers that can be cured.

The following editorial comment concerning an article on treatment stratification based upon risk that was published in the February 2018 *Journal of Urology* sums up current trends in prostate cancer management:

> **"Low risk patients do not benefit from radical therapy unless perhaps they are exceedingly young. Intermediate risk patients die of prostate cancer and benefit from treatment. High risk patients must be selected carefully for treatment, as many will not benefit given the risk of occult metastatic disease. Most importantly, men have to live long enough to benefit from treatment for treatment to be undertaken. In practice that is the hardest thing to figure out. In many regards, this study is reassuring in that it supports the current trends in urological oncology, i.e., surveillance for low risk patients, early intervention for intermediate risk cancers in young patients and strides towards multimodal therapy to improve outcomes in patients with high risk disease."**
> **—Dr. Samir S. Taneja, Professor of Urological Oncology, NYU Langone Medical Center**

The following are the sage words of Dr. Willet Whitmore from 1973. He served as chief of urology at what is now Memorial Sloan-Kettering Cancer Center and died in 1995 of prostate cancer:

> **"Appropriate treatment implies that therapy be applied neither to those patients for whom it is unnecessary nor to those for whom it will prove**

ineffective. Furthermore, the therapy should be that which will most assuredly permit the individual a qualitatively and quantitatively normal life. It need not necessarily involve an effort at cancer cure. Human nature in physicians, be they surgeons, radiotherapists, or medical oncologists, is apt to attribute good results following treatment to such treatment and bad results to the cancer, ignoring what is sometimes the equally plausible possibility that the good results are as much a consequence of the natural history of the tumor as are the bad results."

—Dr. Willet Whitmore

Chapter 4: What is the Prostate?

The prostate gland is a mysterious male reproductive organ that can be a source of curiosity, anxiety, fear and potential trouble. Since this gland is a midline organ nestled deep within the pelvis, I like to think of it as man's "center of gravity."

PROSTATE AND SEMINAL VESICLES

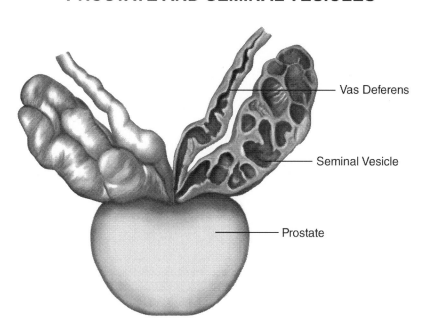

Figure 1. Prostate And Seminal Vesicles

The prostate functions to produce prostate fluid, a milky liquid that is a nutrient and energy vehicle for sperm. Like the breast in many respects, the prostate consists of numerous glands that produce this fluid and ducts that convey the fluid. At the time of sexual climax, prostate smooth muscle squeezes prostatic fluid out of the glands through the prostate ducts and into the urethra (channel that runs from the bladder to the tip of the penis that conducts urine and semen); here it mixes with secretions from the other male reproductive organs—fluid from the seminal vesicles, which constitutes the bulk of the volume of the semen, as well as with sperm from the testes—to form semen.

MALE PELVIC ORGANS

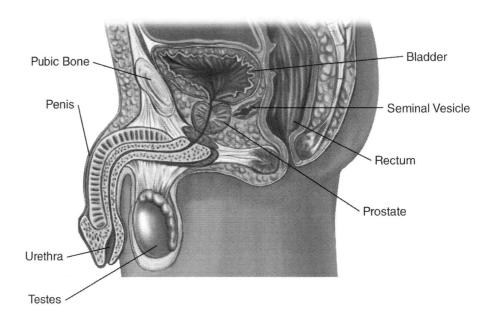

Figure 2. Male Pelvic Organs

The prostate gland is located behind the pubic bone and is attached to the bladder above and the urethra below. The rectum is directly behind the prostate (which permits access for prostate exam). The prostate is situated at the crossroads of the urinary and reproductive tracts and completely en-

velops the urethra, enabling its many ducts to drain into the urethra. However, this necessary anatomical relationship between the prostate and the
urethra can potentially be the source of many issues for the aging male. A
young man's prostate is about the size of a walnut, but under the influence
of aging, genetics and the male hormone testosterone, the prostate gradually increases in size. As it does so, it can compress and obstruct the urethra,
giving rise to bothersome urinary symptoms.

PROSTATE ZONES

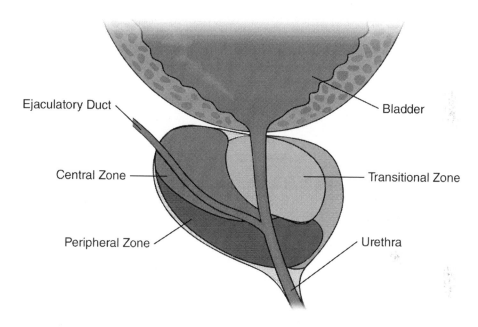

Figure 3. Prostate Zones

The prostate gland is comprised of different anatomical zones. Most cancers originate in the "peripheral zone" at the back of the prostate, which can
be accessed via digital rectal exam. The "transition zone" surrounds the
urethra and is the site where benign enlargement of the prostate occurs.
The "central zone" surrounds the ejaculatory ducts, which run from the

seminal vesicles to the urethra. The prostate is enclosed by a capsule composed of collagen, elastin and smooth muscle.

Curious Facts About the Prostate

- The function of the prostate is to produce a milky fluid that is a nutrient vehicle for sperm.

- Prostate "massage" is sometimes done by urologists to "milk" the prostate to obtain a specimen for laboratory analysis.

- The prostate undergoes an initial growth spurt at puberty and a second one starting at age 40 or so.

- Under the influence of aging, genetics and testosterone, the prostate gland often enlarges and constricts the urethra, which can cause annoying urinary symptoms.

- In the absence of testosterone, the prostate never develops.

- The prostate consists of 70% glands and 30% muscle. Prostate muscle fibers contract at sexual climax to squeeze prostate fluid into the urethra. Excessive prostate muscle tone, often stress-related, can give rise to the same urinary symptoms that are caused by benign enlargement of the prostate.

- Women have a female version of the prostate, known as the Skene's glands.

Chapter 5: His Prostate and Her Breasts

Although not particularly relevant to learning about prostate cancer, the following digression, nonetheless, is an interesting comparison of the prostate and mammary glands, which have many more similarities than differences.

The male prostate and the female breasts are both sources of fascination, curiosity, and fear. Surprisingly, they have much in common. Hidden deep in the pelvis at the crossroads of the male urinary and reproductive systems, the prostate is arguably man's center of gravity. On the other hand, the breasts—with an equal aura of mystique and power—are situated in the chest superficial to the pectorals, contributing to the alluring female form and allowing ready access for the hungry infant, oddly an erogenous zone as well as a feeding zone.

The breasts and prostate both serve important "nutritional" roles. Each function to manufacture a milky white fluid; in the case of the breasts, the milk serving as nourishment for infants, and in the case of the prostate, the "milk" serving as sustenance for sperm cells.

Breasts are composed of glandular tissue that produces milk and ducts that transport the milk to the nipple. The remainder of the breast consists of fatty tissue. The glandular tissue is sustained by the sex hormone estrogen and after menopause, when estrogen levels decline, the glandular tissue withers, with the fatty tissue predominating.

The prostate is made up of glandular tissue that produces prostate "milk" and ducts that empty into the urethra. At the time of ejaculation, the prostate fluid mixes with other reproductive secretions and sperm to form semen. The remainder of the prostate consists of fibro-muscular tissue. The glandular tissue is sustained by the sex hormone testosterone and after age 40 there is a slow and gradual increase in the size of the prostate gland because of glandular and fibro-muscular cell growth.

Access to the breasts as mammary feeding zones is via stimulation of the erect nipples through the act of nursing. Access to prostate fluid is via stimulation of the erect penis, with the release of semen and its prostate fluid component at the time of ejaculation.

The breasts and prostate can be considered reproductive organs since they are vital to the nourishment of infants and sperm, respectively. At the same time they are sexual organs. The breasts have a dual role that not only provide milk to infants, but also function as erogenous zones that attract the interest of the opposite sex and contribute positively to the sexual and thus, reproductive process. Similarly, the prostate is both a reproductive and sexual organ, since sexual stimulation resulting in ejaculation is the means of accessing the prostate's reproductive function.

Both breast and prostate are susceptible to similar disease processes including infection, inflammation and cancer. Congestion of the breast and prostate glands can result in a painful mastitis and prostatitis, respectively. Excluding skin cancer, prostate cancer is the most common cancer in men and breast cancer is the most common cancer in women. Breast and prostate tissue are dependent upon the sex hormones estrogen and testosterone, respectively, and one mode of treatment for both breast cancer and prostate cancer is suppression of these hormones with medications. Both breast and prostate cancer incidence increase with aging. The median age of breast cancer at diagnosis is the early 60s and breast cancer is the second most common form of cancer death, after lung cancer. There are about 3 million breast cancer survivors in the USA. The median age of prostate cancer at diagnosis is the mid-late 60s and prostate cancer is the second most common form of cancer death, after lung cancer. There are about 3 million prostate cancer survivors in the USA.

Both breast and prostate cancer are often detected during screening examinations before symptoms have developed. Breast cancer is often picked up via screening mammography, whereas prostate cancer is often identified via an elevated or accelerated PSA blood test. Alternatively, breast and prostate cancer are detected when an abnormal lump is found on breast exam or digital rectal exam of the prostate, respectively.

Both breast and prostate cells may develop a non-invasive form of cancer known as carcinoma-in-situ—ductal carcinoma-in-situ (DCIS) and high-grade prostate intraepithelial neoplasia (HGPIN), respectively—non-invasive forms in which the abnormal cells have not grown beyond the layer of cells where they originated, often predating invasive cancer by years.

Family history is relevant to both breast and prostate cancer since there can be a genetic predisposition to both types and having a first degree relative with the disease will typically increase one's risk. Both women and men can inherit abnormal BRCA1 and BRCA2 tumor suppressor genes. Women who inherit BRCA1 and BRCA2 abnormal genes have about a 60% and 45% chance of developing breast cancer by age 70, respectively. Men who inherit the BRCA1 abnormal gene have a slightly increased risk for prostate cancer; men who inherit the BRCA2 abnormal gene have about a seven-fold increased risk. BRCA1 mutations double the risk of metastatic prostate cancer and BRCA2 mutations increase the risk of metastatic prostate cancer by 4-6 times, with earlier onset and higher grade at diagnosis.

Imaging tests used in the diagnosis and evaluation of both breast and prostate cancers are similar with ultrasonography and MRI commonly used. Treatment modalities for both breast and prostate cancer share much in common with important roles for surgery, radiation, chemotherapy and hormone therapy.

Chapter 6: What is the Digital Rectal Examination (DRE)?

This is not a fancy and sophisticated, high-tech "digital" as opposed to "analog" test. A DRE is an important part of the male physical exam in which a gloved and lubricated examining index finger (digit) is placed gently in the patient's rectum to feel the surface of the prostate and gain valuable information about its health. After age 40, an annual DRE of the prostate is highly recommended.

DIGITAL RECTAL EXAM

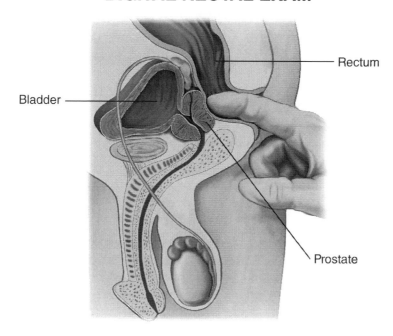

Figure 4. Digital Rectal Exam

Although it is not a particularly pleasant examination, it is brief and not painful. Urologists do not relish doing this exam any more than patients like receiving it, but it provides essential information that cannot be derived by any other means. If the prostate has an abnormal consistency, a hardness, lump, bump, or simply feels uneven and asymmetrical, it may be a sign of prostate cancer.

When teaching medical students, urologists often use hand anatomy to explain DRE of the prostate. Turn your hand so that the palm is up and make a fist. The normal prostate feels like the spongy, muscular, fleshy tissue at the base of the thumb, whereas cancer feels hard, like the knuckle of the thumb.

DRE in conjunction with the PSA blood test is the best means of screening for prostate cancer. Detection rates for prostate cancer are highest when using both tests, followed by PSA alone, followed by DRE alone.

The pathological features of prostate cancers detected on an abnormal DRE are, in general, less favorable than those of cancers detected by a PSA elevation. In other words, if the cancer can be felt, we tend to worry about it more than if it cannot be felt, as it is often at a more advanced stage.

Fact: The PSA blood test is NOT a substitute for the DRE. Both tests provide valuable and complementary information about your prostate health.

Chapter 7: What is the PSA Test?

PSA (Prostate Specific Antigen) is a protein produced by cells of the prostate gland. PSA is an enzyme known as a protease that functions to liquefy semen following sexual intercourse and ejaculation, which aids the transit of the sperm cells to the egg.

The PSA blood test was FDA (Food and Drug Administration) approved in 1994 and remains the best tool currently available for detecting prostate cancer in its earliest— and most curable—stages. Although PSA is widely accepted as a tumor marker, it is prostate organ-specific but not cancer-specific. In other words, PSA can be elevated due to benign conditions besides from prostate cancer, including prostatitis (inflammation of the prostate) and benign prostatic hyperplasia (BPH, an enlargement of the prostate gland). PSA gradually increases with the aging process in accordance with the enlarging prostate gland that occurs with growing older.

Prostate cancer cells do not make more PSA than normal prostate cells. The elevated PSA detected in the blood of prostate cancer patients occurs because of a disruption of the cellular structure of the prostate cells. The loss of this structural barrier allows accelerated leakage of PSA from the prostate into the blood circulation. Similarly, a PSA leak from disrupted prostate cells can occur with BPH, prostatitis, and prostate manipulation (a vigorous prostate examination or a prostate biopsy).

PSA is arguably the best tumor marker in all disciplines of medicine and provides an excellent means of monitoring men already diagnosed with prostate cancer who have been treated or are being managed with active surveillance. Rising PSA levels after treatment may be the first sign of cancer recurrence. Such a "biochemical" relapse typically precedes "clinical" relapse by months or years. However, a single accelerated PSA level in a patient with a history of prostate cancer does not always mean cancer recurrence. A trend of rising PSA over time is much more informative than is a single elevated PSA.

PSA screening is far from perfect, fraught with false negatives (presence of prostate cancer in men with low PSA) and false positives (absence of prostate cancer in men with high PSA). The most informative use of PSA screening is serially, with comparison on a year-to-year basis providing meaningful information, much more so than a single, out-of-context PSA. Because PSA values can fluctuate from lab to lab, it is always a good idea to attempt to use the same laboratory for the testing.

Statistically, about 90% of men have a normal PSA. Of the 10% of men with an elevated PSA, about 30% will have prostate cancer and 70% will have benign pathology on biopsy. Despite its limitations, PSA testing has substantially reduced both the incidence of metastatic disease and the death rate from prostate cancer.

PSA testing should not be thought of as a stand-alone test, but rather as part of a comprehensive approach to early prostate cancer detection. Baseline PSA testing for men in their 40s is useful for predicting the future potential for prostate cancer.

Fact: At the 2018 American Urology Meeting in San Francisco, Dr. David Crawford gave a "State of the Art" lecture entitled "PSA 1.5 is the New 4.0." In a study of 350,000 men with a mean age of 55, median PSA was 1.0. Those with a PSA < 1.5 had a 0.5% risk of developing prostate cancer, those between 1.5-4.0 had about an 8% risk, and those > 4.0 had greater than a 10% risk. He recommended that men with a PSA < 1.5 do not need a repeat PSA for 5 years and that a PSA of > 1.5 should be the new cutoff point (as opposed to the traditional 4.0 cutoff point), not necessarily triggering a biopsy, but for prompting further clinical tests and biomarkers to select patients who need a more critical evaluation.

The age at which to stop screening needs to be individualized, since "functional" age trumps "chronological" age and there are men 75 years old and older who are in phenomenal shape, have a greater than 10-year life expectancy and should be offered screening. This population of older men may certainly benefit from the early diagnosis of aggressive prostate cancer that has the potential to destroy quantity and quality of life. However, if a man is elderly and has medical issues and a life expectancy of less than 10 years, there is little sense in screening. Another important factor is individual preference since the decision to screen should be a collaborative decision between patient and physician.

Fact: Most urologists do not believe in screening or treating men who have a life expectancy of less than 10 years. This is because prostate cancer rarely causes death in the first decade after diagnosis and other competing medical issues often will do so before the prostate cancer has a chance to. Prostate cancer is generally a slow-growing process and early detection and treatment is directed at extending life well beyond the decade following diagnosis.

Advantages of PSA testing:

• A normal result can put one's mind at ease.

• An elevated or accelerated PSA that leads to prostate biopsy and diagnosis of cancer most often finds prostate cancer in its earliest and most treatable state. Those at greatest risk can be managed appropriately (surgery or radiation) and many cured, avoiding the potential for progression of cancer and devastating consequences, including painful metastases and death.

• PSA is unquestionably the best marker (to gauge prostate cancer status) in the follow-up of men who have been treated for prostate cancer by any means.

Disadvantages of PSA testing:

• Prostate cancer may be present even with a normal PSA.

• An elevated PSA does not always mean prostate cancer.

• An elevated PSA often leads to other invasive tests that may end up being normal.

• A PSA elevation may reveal low grade cancers that never require treatment.

Refinements in PSA Testing

<u>PSA Velocity</u> Comparing the PSA values year to year is most informative. Generally, PSA will increase by only a small increment, reflecting benign prostate growth. If PSA accelerates at a greater rate than anticipated—a condition known as accelerated PSA velocity—further evaluation is indicated.

27

Fact: An isolated PSA (out of context) is not particularly helpful. What is meaningful is comparing PSA on a year-to-year basis and observing for any acceleration above and beyond the expected annual incremental change associated with aging and benign prostate growth. Many labs use a PSA of 4.0 as a cutoff for abnormal, so it is possible that one can be falsely lulled into the impression that their PSA is normal. For example, if the PSA is 1.0 and a year later it is 3.0, it is still considered a "normal" PSA (because it is less than 4.0) even though it has tripled (highly suspicious for a problem) and mandates further investigation.

PSA Density PSA density (PSA divided by prostate volume) is the PSA level corrected to the size of the prostate. The prostate volume can be determined by imaging studies including ultrasound or MRI. PSA elevations are less worrisome under the circumstance of an enlarged prostate. A PSA density > 0.15 is concerning for prostate cancer.

Fact: The prostate can be considered a "factory" that produces a product called PSA; the larger the factory, the higher the expected PSA.

Free/Total PSA PSA circulates in the blood in two forms: a "free" form in which the PSA is unbound, and a "complex" PSA in which the PSA is bound to a protein. The free PSA/total PSA ratio can offer a predictive value (similar to how HDL cholesterol/total cholesterol can be helpful in a person with an elevated cholesterol level). The higher the free to total PSA ratio, the greater the chance that benign enlargement of the prostate is the underlying source of the PSA elevation. In men with a PSA between 4 and 10, the probability of cancer is 9-16% if the free/total PSA ratio is greater than 25%; 18-30% if the ratio is 19-25%; 27-41% if the ratio is 11-18%, and the probability of cancer increases to 49-65% if the ratio is less than 10%.

The PSA Controversy

Prostate cancer screening with PSA has been the subject of intense controversy and debate, one that I never quite understood. A major backlash against screening occurred in 2012 with the United States Preventive Services Task Force (USPSTF) grade "D" recommendation against PSA screening and their call for total abandonment of the test. This organization counseled against the use of PSA testing in healthy men, postulating that the test does not save lives and leads to more tests and treatments that needlessly cause pain, incontinence and erectile dysfunction. Of note, there was not a single urologist on the committee. The same organization had previously advised that women in their 40s not undergo routine mammography, setting off another blaze of controversy. Uncertainty in the lay press prompted both patients and physicians to question PSA testing and recommendations for prostate biopsy. Sadly, in the aftermath of the USPSTF recommendations against PSA screening, there has been a spike of men with higher PSA levels and more aggressive prostate cancer.

Is there really any harm in screening? Although there are potential side effects from prostate biopsy (although they are few and far between) and there certainly are potential side effects with treatment, there are no side effects from drawing a small amount of blood.

My take: When interpreted appropriately, the PSA test provides valuable information in the diagnosis, pre-treatment staging, risk assessment and monitoring of prostate cancer patients. Marginalizing this important test does a great disservice to patients who may benefit from early prostate cancer detection.

PSA screening has resulted in detecting prostate cancer in earlier and more curable stages, before it has a chance to spread and potentially becomes incurable. PSA screening has unequivocally reduced metastatic prostate cancer and death from prostate cancer: USA death rates from prostate cancer have fallen 4% annually since 1992, five years after introduction of PSA testing. Unfortunately, rigid guidelines do not allow for a nuanced and individualized approach to early prostate cancer detection. Although PSA has many shortcomings, when used intelligently and appropriately, it will continue to save lives.

Fact: I have practiced urology in both the pre-PSA and the post-PSA era. In my early career (pre-PSA era), it was not uncommon to be called to the emergency room to consult on men who could not urinate, who on digital rectal exam were found to have rock-hard prostate glands and imaging studies that showed diffuse spread of prostate cancer to their bones—metastatic prostate cancer with a grim prognosis. Fortunately, in the current era, that scenario occurs extremely infrequently because of PSA screening. These days, most men who present with metastatic disease are those who have not had PSA screening as part of their annual physical exams.

Fact: 95% of male urologists and 80% of primary care physicians older than 50 have PSA screening—clearly those in the know feel that screening is beneficial.

"PSA is the best screening test we have for prostate cancer, and until there is a replacement for PSA, it would be unconscionable to stop it. Contrary to the USPSTF report, compelling evidence shows that PSA screening reduces prostate cancer deaths. This evidence needs to be shared with the public."

—Dr. William Catalona, Professor of Urology, Feinberg Northwestern School of Medicine

"Treatment or non-treatment decisions can be made once the cancer is found, but not knowing about it in the first place surely burns bridges."

—Dr. Joseph A. Smith, Professor of Urology, Vanderbilt School of Medicine, Editor, Journal of Urology

"We need to separate screening from treatment and screen smarter. The potential side effects of treatment should not influence the diagnosis of prostate cancer by the proper means."

—Dr. Judd Moul, Professor of Urology, Duke University School of Medicine

30

Chapter 8: What is Prostate MRI (Magnetic Resonance Imaging)?

Multi-parametric MRI is a high-resolution imaging test that is an important tool for prostate cancer diagnosis, targeting of biopsies, clinical staging, surgical planning, follow-up of prostate cancer patients managed with active surveillance and in the evaluation of recurrent prostate cancer following treatment. MRI uses a powerful magnet to enable viewing of the prostate gland and surrounding tissues in multiple planes of view without requiring radiation. It allows for the identification of areas suspicious for cancer and the ability to perform "targeted" biopsies as opposed to "systematic" biopsies. Although useful in the diagnostic evaluation of any man who has a suspicion of prostate cancer, it is particularly beneficial in men who have had previous benign prostate biopsies who have persistent PSA elevations or accelerations.

MRI is a valuable part of the diagnostic armamentarium, increasing the detection rate of clinically significant (higher grade) prostate cancers, while reducing the detection rate of clinically insignificant (lower grade) cancers. MRI provides anatomical details about the neurovascular bundles, urinary bladder, seminal vesicles, pelvic lymph nodes, bowel loops and pelvic bones and beneficial staging information on tumor extension beyond the prostate capsule, pelvic lymph node enlargement and seminal vesicle involvement.

Prostate MRI is performed at specialty imaging centers. Preparation involves a Fleet enema to clear gas from the rectum that can generate artifacts on the MRI images making interpretation suboptimal. A coil placed in the rectum (endorectal coil) is no longer necessary as it was in prior versions of MRI. The study is done before and after the injection of intravenous contrast to optimize the results. MRI cannot be performed under the following circumstances: presence of pacemaker, recent coronary artery stent placement, ferromagnetic brain aneurysm clips and the presence of metal near the spinal cord, e.g., bullet fragments.

The value of prostate MRI is highly operator-dependent and requires a quality study and interpretation by a skilled and experienced radiologist. Sophisticated software performs image analysis, assisting radiologists in interpreting and scoring MRI results. A validated scoring system known as PI-RADS (Prostate Imaging Reporting and Data System) is used. This scoring system helps urologists make decisions about whether to biopsy the prostate and, if so, how to optimize the biopsy.

PI-RADS	Definition
I	most probably benign (clinically significant cancer highly unlikely)
II	probably benign (clinically significant cancer unlikely)
III	indeterminate (clinically significant cancer equivocal)
IV	probably cancer (clinically significant cancer likely)
V	most probably cancer (clinically significant cancer highly likely)

MRI is by no means infallible, as clinically significant cancers (particularly small ones) are not always apparent on MRI, and PIRADS-4 and PIRADS-5 lesions when biopsied are not always found to contain clinically significant cancers. An additional concern is its expense. Some urologists believe in obtaining a prostate MRI on all patients prior to performing a prostate biopsy, whereas others reserve MRI for patients with a previous negative biopsy in the face of a rising PSA. In the former setting, a biopsy remains the only definitive means of assessment regardless of the PIRADS score, one of the key utilities of the MRI being to help precisely target the biopsy. However, in the latter setting, when the MRI reading is PIRADS-1 or PIRADS-2, a repeat biopsy can often be avoided.

Fact: PSA, DRE and MRI are all useful and informative tests, but the prostate biopsy (tissue sampling) is the only way to know for sure if one has prostate cancer. In other words, whereas PSA, DRE and MRI are "suggestive," the biopsy is "definitive." "The buck stops here" applies to the biopsy.

Chapter 9: What is an Ultrasound-Guided Prostate Biopsy?

If there is concern or suspicion for prostate cancer—most commonly based upon an elevation in PSA, an accelerated PSA velocity, or an abnormal digital rectal exam—the definitive diagnostic test is an ultrasound-guided prostate biopsy. The other reasons for prostate biopsy are to reevaluate pre-cancerous lesions, including high grade prostate intra-epithelial neoplasia (HGPIN) and atypical small acinar proliferation (ASAP), for monitoring patients on active surveillance and in the evaluation of men who have received prostate cancer treatment who have a rising PSA. To reiterate, although DRE, PSA, and MRI are suggestive and helpful, it is the biopsy that is definitive.

Prostate ultrasound is an effective means of prostate imaging using sound waves (like sonar on a submarine) generated by an ultrasound probe placed in the rectum. Reflected echoes create a high-resolution image of the prostate to measure the prostate volume, check for abnormalities, and precisely guide the biopsies. The ultrasound image alone is not sufficient to diagnose prostate cancer without a tissue biopsy. MRI is often used prior to the biopsy to see if there are any discrete abnormalities that need to be targeted, as opposed to systematic biopsies, which are biopsies of the different regions of the prostate.

Preparation for ultrasound-guided prostate biopsy involves a Fleet enema the evening before the biopsy to cleanse the rectum, discontinuing any anti-coagulant medications and blood thinners for a week or so prior to the procedure and oral antibiotics to be taken prior to the biopsy, since the biopsies are performed via the rectum.

The prostate biopsy can be performed using a local anesthetic or, alternatively, with intravenous sedation. I prefer to do the biopsies in the office setting using intravenous sedation provided by an anesthesiologist, which makes the experience more pleasant for the patient and avoids the need for local anesthesia injections into the prostate, which can increase the risk of infection. Two antibiotics are administered intravenously immediately prior to the biopsy.

The ultrasound/biopsy is about a 10-15 minute procedure, although you will need to arrive 30 minutes prior to and remain for about 30 minutes after the procedure. In the knee-chest position while lying on your side, the ultra-sound probe is gently placed into the rectum. After obtaining imaging and volume measurements, prostate biopsies are obtained with a spring-driven needle device that is passed through the needle guide attached to the ultra-sound probe. Generally, a minimum of 12 biopsies are obtained—six from each side with two biopsies each from the apex, mid-gland and base, provid-ing a pathological "map" of the prostate. Each biopsy is placed in a separate specimen container noting the site of the biopsy and is carefully examined by a skilled pathologist to make a diagnosis.

If an abnormality is visualized on ultrasound—classically a hypo-echoic re-gion (an area with less echoes than adjacent prostate tissue)—this specific area will be biopsied as well. Often, MRI is performed prior to the biopsy and any specific areas of suspicion identified on MRI are matched with the ultrasound and targeted biopsies are obtained of these areas, as well as the standard 12 mapping biopsies. MRI/ultrasound fusion-guided biopsy is a means of fusing pre-biopsy MRI prostate imaging with ultrasound-guided prostate biopsy images in real time, so that the suspicious regions seen on MRI can be precisely targeted. Fusion-guided biopsies require sophisticated hardware and software technology and the combined efforts of the radiolo-gist, technician and urologist. Alternatively, cognitive-guided biopsies are ultrasound-guided biopsies performed while simultaneously viewing the pre-biopsy MRI images to target the regions of concern.

After the biopsy, it is important to stay well hydrated, complete the pre-scribed antibiotics, and to take it easy for a day or so. Blood in the urine or stool following a biopsy is common and typically resolves within a few days or so. It is not uncommon to experience blood in the semen for up to 6 weeks after the biopsy. It generally takes 7-10 days or so to receive the biopsy results.

Trans-perineal (via the anatomical region between scrotum and anus) map-ping prostate biopsies are sometimes done as an alternative to the trans-rectal biopsy described above. Ultrasound is used to image the prostate and numerous mapping biopsies—typically at 5 mm intervals—are done via a perineal template. This provides a pathological map of the entire prostate, sometimes used to obtain a primary biopsy but more often used as a confirmatory biopsy that improves staging because of the number of biopsies obtained at precise anatomical locations.

Chapter 10: What Will My Biopsy Report Tell Me?

There are four possible outcomes of the prostate biopsy:

• Benign prostate tissue

• HGPIN (High Grade Prostate Intraepithelial Neoplasia)

• ASAP (Atypical Small Acinar Proliferation)

• Prostate Cancer

Prostate Histology 101

The prostate gland is divided into anatomical subdivisions known as lobes. The prostate is organized like a tree with a major trunk draining each lobe, each trunk served by many ducts which progressively branch out into smaller and smaller ducts. At the end of each duct is an acinus (Latin, meaning *berry*), analogous to a leaf at the end of a tree branch. Each acinus is lined by cells that secrete prostate fluid, a nutrient vehicle for sperm that is an important component of semen. Each acinus is surrounded by a basement membrane that separates the secretory cells from surrounding structures.

What is HGPIN?

HGPIN is an acronym for "High Grade Prostate Intraepithelial Neoplasia." HGPIN occurs in 0.6 - 24% of biopsies. It is a microscopic abnormality marked by an abnormal appearance and proliferation of cells within ducts and acini, but the abnormal cells do not extend beyond the basement membrane to other parts of the prostate (as occurs with prostate cancer). HGPIN is considered a pre-malignant precursor lesion to prostate cancer.

Current recommendations for men who are found to have one site of HGPIN are to follow-up as one would follow for a benign biopsy, with annual digital rectal exam and PSA. However, if there are multiple biopsies indicating HGPIN (multifocal HGPIN), a repeat biopsy is recommended in 6-12 months, with focused sampling of identified areas and adjacent sites. The more cores containing HGPIN on an initial prostate biopsy, the greater the likelihood of cancer on subsequent biopsies. The risk for prostate cancer following the diagnosis of multifocal HGPIN is about 25%.

What is ASAP?

ASAP is an acronym for "Atypical Small Acinar Proliferation." ASAP occurs in 5 - 20% of biopsies. It is a microscopic abnormality marked by a collection of prostate acini that are suspicious but not diagnostic for prostate cancer, falling below the diagnostic "threshold." The risk for cancer following the diagnosis of ASAP on re-biopsy is approximately 40%. It is recommended that men with ASAP should undergo re-biopsy within 3 to 6 months, with focused sampling of identified areas and adjacent sites.

What is Prostate Cancer?

Prostate cancer is a microscopic abnormality marked by an abnormal appearance and proliferation of cells within prostate ducts and acini that have broken through the basement membrane barrier to involve the deep tissues of the prostate. The appearance of prostate cancer cells and their patterns of growth differ from normal cells in ways that enable the pathologist to recognize and diagnose the biopsy as cancer. The degree to which these tissues demonstrate malignancy allows the pathologist to assign a grade to the cancerous tissue. The higher the grade, the more profound the malignant changes.

If the prostate biopsy demonstrates prostate cancer, the pathologist will provide a detailed report indicating the following:

• Number of cores showing cancer

• Percent of cancer involvement in each core

• Location of the cores with cancer

- Gleason score (the pathologist's numerical quantification of aggressiveness)

- Biopsy map

Most prostate cancers are "adenocarcinomas" (*adeno*—"pertaining to a gland" and *carcinoma*—"a cancer that develops in epithelial cells")—a type of malignancy that originates from glandular cells. On occasion, a prostate adenocarcinoma is found to be an "intraductal carcinoma," a proliferation of malignant prostate cells that fill and distend the inside space of prostatic ducts and acini, with the cells around the basement membrane largely preserved. Intraductal prostate cancer is often invasive, high grade, and typically has large tumor volumes.

Rarely, a prostate cancer is a "small cell carcinoma," a type of malignancy that originates from neuro-endocrine cells. This high grade and aggressive cancer accounts for only about 1% of prostate cancers and is typically diagnosed at an advanced stage, tends to progress rapidly and has a poor prognosis with an average survival of less than one year.

Chapter 11: What is the Gleason Grading System?

Dr. Donald Gleason, the former chief of pathology at the Minneapolis VA Center, devised a prostate cancer grading system many years ago that is still used today. His legacy, the system that he devised and that bears his name —the Gleason score—provides one of the best guides to the prognosis and treatment of an individual case of prostate cancer.

Gleason grade

Gleason grade is determined by the examining pathologist who studies the biopsied prostate tissue under a microscope. Grade is indicative of the extent of difference in the cellular architecture of cancer cells as compared with normal cells. Low grade cancers appear almost like normal cells whereas high grade cancers bear little resemblance to normal cells. Gleason grade range from 3 (just over the threshold for cancer) to 5 (the cells that have the most cancerous appearance). Dr. Gleason determined that prostate cancer grade was the most reliable indicator of the potential for cancer growth and spread.

Gleason score

The cancer from any individual biopsy site is often heterogeneous as opposed to homogeneous. In other words, cancer cells can show various architectural patterns, often a predominant pattern as well as secondary and tertiary patterns. To determine Gleason score, the pathologist assigns a separate numerical grade to the two most predominant architectural patterns of the cancer cells, the first number representing the grade of the primary (most predominant) pattern and the second number representing the grade of the secondary pattern. The sum of the two grades is the Gleason score. The lowest possible score is 6; the highest is 10.

Gleason score predicts the aggressiveness and behavior of the cancer. Higher scores indicate a worse prognosis than lower scores because the more mutated cells typically grow faster than the more normal-appearing ones. Prognosis also depends on further refinements. For example, a Gleason score of 7 can occur two ways: "4+3" or "3+4". With "4+3," cancer cells in the most predominant category appear more aggressive than those in the secondary pattern, suggesting a more serious threat than a "3+4" score, in which cells in the most predominant group appear less aggressive.

Gleason grade groups

There are 5 Gleason grade groups based upon Gleason score:

Grade Group 1 (Gleason score 3+3=6)

Grade Group 2 (Gleason score 3+4=7)

Grade Group 3 (Gleason score 4+3=7)

Grade Group 4 (Gleason score 4+4=8 or 3+5=8 or 5+3= 8)

Grade Group 5 (Gleason score 4+5=9 or 5+4= 9 or 5+5=10)

Chapter 12: What Are Prostate Cancer Biomarkers?

Prostate specific antigen (PSA) was the first prostate cancer biomarker, singularly responsible for revolutionizing the diagnosis and follow-up of prostate cancer. Following surgical removal of the prostate, PSA should become undetectable within a few weeks and following radiation therapy, PSA should gradually decline to its lowest level in about 18-24 months and thereafter remain stable.

There are several new biomarkers that can help with the decision of whether or not to biopsy as well as to inform and support prostate cancer management decisions. These decisions include active surveillance vs. active treatment, the specific means of treatment for early and localized cancer, and when to pursue androgen deprivation therapy (a form of treatment to be discussed in more detail later).

Often more important than histology (the appearance of the cancer under the microscope) is the biology of the prostate cancer. Genomics reveals the biological potential of any given cancer. Indeed, about 15% of low risk prostate cancers have high risk genomic features.

PROSTATE CANCER SCREENING BIOMARKERS

Prostate health index (PHI) This is a compilation of several different PSA sub-types, including pro-PSA, free PSA and total PSA into a single score. It can help discriminate between higher and lower grade disease. PHI score coupled with other factors including age, prostate volume, DRE (abnormal DRE vs. normal DRE) and biopsy history (prior prostate biopsy vs. no prior prostate biopsy) are used to help determine the need for biopsy in a patient with suspected prostate cancer.

Prostate cancer antigen (PCA3) urine test PCA3 is a specific type of RNA (ribonucleic acid) that is released in high levels by prostate cancer cells. Its expression is 60-100 times greater in prostate cancer cells than benign

43

prostate cells, which makes this test much more specific for prostate cancer than PSA. The first ounce of urine voided immediately after prostate massage (a vigorous DRE with the intent of milking the prostate) is rich in prostatic fluid and cells and is collected and tested for the quantity of PCA3 genetic material present. Urinary levels of PCA3 are not affected by prostate enlargement or inflammation, as opposed to PSA levels. PCA3 > 25 is suspicious for prostate cancer.

4Kscore test 4Kscore test measures blood levels of four different prostate-derived proteins: total PSA, free PSA, intact PSA and human kallikrein 2. Levels of these biomarkers are combined with the patient's age, DRE, and history of prior biopsy. These factors are processed using an algorithm to calculate the risk of finding an aggressive prostate cancer (Gleason score 7 or higher) if a prostate biopsy were to be performed. The test can increase the accuracy of prostate cancer diagnosis, particularly in its most aggressive forms. It cannot be used if a patient has had a DRE in the previous 4 days, nor can it be used if one has taken finasteride (Proscar) or dutasteride (Avodart) within the previous six months. Additionally, it cannot be used in patients who have undergone any procedure to treat symptomatic prostate enlargement or any invasive urologic procedure in the prior 6 months.

Apifiny test This test measures the immune response to prostate cancer, detecting autoantibody proteins in the blood that are produced against prostate cancer cells. It is a risk assessment tool that does not rely on PSA. A score of 1-100 is given: the higher the score, the greater the chance for the presence of prostate cancer.

BIOMARKER TO CONFIRM A NEGATIVE BIOPSY

ConfirmMDx Since a biopsy of the prostate samples only a small volume of the total prostate, it is possible to have benign biopsy results when in fact an underlying cancer was missed. This particular assay is done on prostate tissue derived from a negative biopsy to help determine its accuracy. It quantitates the chemical status of certain genes to detect abnormal changes associated with the presence of prostate cancer. ConfirmMDx detects a "halo" associated with the presence of cancer at the DNA level, which may be detected in prostate cancer tissue despite a normal microscopic appearance. This test helps identify low risk men who may forego a repeat biopsy and high risk men who would benefit from a repeat biopsy.

BIOMARKERS TO PREDICT RECURRENCE AFTER PROSTATECTOMY

Prolaris (cell cycle progression score) This assay uses prostate cancer tissue derived from prostatectomy to calculate a score based upon RNA-expression levels of 31 genes to help predict cancer aggressiveness, risk of a rising PSA, and risk of death from prostate cancer.

Decipher (prostate cancer genomic classifier) This assay measures the expression levels of numerous RNA biomarkers in prostate cancer tissue to create a probability model to predict the risk of metastases within 5 years of prostatectomy in patients with high risk prostate cancer.

BIOMARKERS TO PREDICT PROGRESSION DURING ACTIVE SURVEILLANCE

These biomarkers use genomic analysis of cancer tissue derived from the biopsy to help predict progressive disease that will require the need for active intervention in men on active surveillance.

Oncotype DX (genomic prostate score) This assay uses prostate cancer tissue to determine the expression of 17 genes, reporting the results using a 100-unit score. The higher the score, the greater the risk for aggressive prostate cancer. The test is useful for men with newly diagnosed prostate cancer to aid in making an informed decision regarding management, specifically to help guide who will benefit from active surveillance vs. who would benefit from surgery or radiation. It is beneficial for men with Gleason score 6 (3+3) and 7 (3+4).

The combination of Gleason score and genomic prostate score is the best predictor of aggressive prostate cancer. A genomic prostate score of < 20 is rarely associated with the potential for metastatic disease or death.

Prolaris (cell cycle progression score) In addition to its use to predict recurrence after prostatectomy, this assay is also useful to predict progression during active surveillance. Prostate cancer tissue is used to calculate a score based upon RNA-expression levels of 31 genes to help predict cancer aggressiveness, risk of a rising PSA, and risk of death from prostate cancer.

ProMark This test uses biopsy material to predict the risk of patients with Gleason score 6 (3+3) or 7 (3+4) of having aggressive prostate cancer using a quantitative analysis of 8 protein biomarkers.

PTEN/TMPRSS2:ERG PTEN (phosphatase and tensin homolog) and ERG (ETS-related gene) mutations are two of the most common mutations found in prostate cancer and tend to occur in conjunction with one another. This molecular test can help predict prostate cancer aggressiveness in patients with Gleason score 6 (3+3) or 7 (3+4) as well as those with HGPIN and ASAP. PTEN is a tumor suppressor gene that if deleted (not present) can indicate the potential for aggressive cancer. TMPRSS2 and ERG are genes that when found to be rearranged from their normal locations and in contact with each other can signify aggressive cancer.

Chapter 13: How is Prostate Cancer Risk Assessed?

RISK STRATIFICATION

Every prostate cancer has a unique biological behavior and a variable potential for progression, spread and death. To determine the most appropriate and effective management strategy, newly diagnosed prostate cancer patients are "risk stratified" to predict the potential for aggressiveness and severity.

Classification of prostate cancer into risk categories is based upon tumor category, Gleason score, volume of cancer on biopsy, PSA, PSA density, and genomic testing. Additional factors that influence treatment choices for prostate cancer are: age and life expectancy, general health status, urinary symptoms and personal preferences.

The extent of prostate cancer—whether localized, regionally advanced or metastatic—is an important factor that informs treatment. Prostatectomy or radiation therapy is appropriate for localized disease, but not so for metastatic disease. Extent or "staging" is determined by digital rectal exam and magnetic resonance imaging; additionally, computerized tomography and bone scan are often obtained when staging unfavorable intermediate risk, high risk or very high risk prostate cancer.

Tumor category

The **TNM** (Tumor/Lymph Nodes/Metastases) system is used to determine the stage of prostate cancer. **T** refers to tumor size; **N** the extent of lymph node involvement; and **M** to the presence or absence of metastasis (spread).

Prostate cancer diagnosed because of a PSA elevation without the presence of an abnormality on DRE is a different tumor category than one diagnosed because of an abnormality on DRE. This is because the presence of palpable cancer (one that can be felt on DRE) indicates that the cancer is already

47

close to the capsule—perhaps beyond the capsule—whereas non-palpable cancer is typically earlier in the natural course of cancer progression.

STAGES OF PROSTATE CANCER

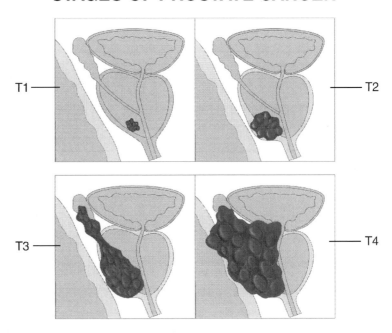

Figure 5. Stages Of Prostate Cancer

Stage T1

Tumor is microscopic and confined to the prostate and not apparent on DRE. T1a is tumor found incidentally in prostate tissue removed because of symptomatic enlargement (< 5 % of prostate tissue removed); T1b is tumor found incidentally in prostate tissue removed because of symptomatic en-largement (> 5 % of prostate tissue removed); T1c is tumor identified by biopsy because of PSA elevation or acceleration.

Stage T2

Tumor is confined to the prostate and is detected by DRE. T2a involves less than half of one side of the prostate; T2b involves more than half of one side; T2c involves both left and right sides of the prostate.

Stage T3 or T4

T3a tumors extend beyond the prostate capsule, sparing the seminal vesicles; T3b tumors invade the seminal vesicles. Stage T4 tumors have spread to organs near the prostate, but within the pelvis, e.g., bladder, rectum or pelvic sidewall.

Stage N+ or M+

Cancer has spread to pelvic lymph nodes (N+) or to lymph nodes, bones, and/or organs distant from the prostate (M+).

Gleason Score

Dr. Gleason devised a clever system that microscopically grades prostate cancer based upon cellular architecture. He recognized that prostate cancer grade is the most reliable indicator of the potential for cancer growth and spread. The grading system that bears his name provides one of the best guides to prognosis and treatment.

To determine Gleason score, the pathologist assigns a separate numerical grade to the two most predominant architectural patterns of the cancer cells, the first number representing the grade of the primary (most predominant) pattern and the second number representing the grade of the secondary pattern. The grades range from 3 (just over the threshold for cancer) to 5 (the cells that have the most cancerous appearance). The sum of the two grades is the Gleason score. The lowest possible score is 6; the highest is 10. The Gleason score predicts the aggressiveness and behavior of the cancer, with higher scores having a worse prognosis than lower scores.

Gleason score is one of the most important factors to be considered prior to making an informed treatment choice. Whereas men with low Gleason scores are often candidates for active surveillance, a high Gleason score mandates more aggressive management.

There are 5 Gleason Grade Groups based upon Gleason score:

Grade Group 1 (Gleason score 3+3=6)

Grade Group 2 (Gleason score 3+4=7)

Grade Group 3 (Gleason score 4+3=7)

Grade Group 4 (Gleason score 4+4=8 or 3+5=8 or 5+3=8)

Grade Group 5 (Gleason score 4+5=9 or 5+4= 9 or 5+5=10)

To help understand the significance of the Gleason score, the rates of undetectable PSA five years after surgical removal of the prostate in Grade Groups 1-5 are the following: 96%, 88%, 63%, 48%, and 26%, respectively.

Number cores with cancer

Generally, at least 12 biopsy cores are obtained and the number of cores that have cancer can provide invaluable information to help guide treatment. The more cores that contain cancer, the greater the volume of cancer and the greater the risk. A man who has 12/12 cores with cancer has a very different disease than a man with 1/12 cores with cancer.

Percent tumor involvement (PTI)

The percentage of cancer in each cancer core is also useful information. In general, the greater the PTI, the greater the risk. A man with cancer in 3/12 cores that involves 100% of each core has a very different disease than a man with cancer in 3/12 cores that involves 5% of each core.

PSA and PSA velocity

PSA is a superb tumor marker for men with prostate cancer. In general, the lower the PSA, the greater the chance of localized (organ-confined) cancer and conversely, the higher the PSA, the greater the chance of non-localized cancer. The lower the PSA, the greater the likelihood of cure with surgery or radiation therapy. Men with a PSA greater than 20 have a higher risk of locally advanced or metastatic disease and a greater likelihood of failing surgery or radiation therapy.

PSA velocity (rate of change over time) also provides essential prognostic information. A high PSA velocity preceding the diagnosis of prostate cancer is associated with a poorer prognosis.

PSA density (PSAD)

PSAD is the relationship of PSA to the size of the prostate, determined by dividing PSA by the prostate volume. The volume of the prostate is easily determined by ultrasound or by MRI (magnetic resonance imaging). A PSA density > 0.15 is considered to be a higher risk.

Genomic testing

Genomic biomarkers have become an increasingly popular tool to help risk stratification. Oncotype DX (genomic prostate score) is one such assay that determines the expression of 17 genes. It is often used for newly diagnosed Gleason 6 (3+3) and 7 (3+4) cancers to help determine who will benefit from active surveillance vs. surgery or radiation.

Age and life expectancy

The prevailing view accepted among prostate cancer experts is that the more years one has left to live, the greater the likelihood that surgery will provide the greatest chance of achieving that potential. So, if you are 43 years old and in perfect health, the most prudent option is often a radical prostatectomy. On the other hand, if you are elderly and have a less than ten-year life expectancy, you likely will not need any treatment as other more pressing medical issues may cause your demise before the prostate cancer has a chance to.

With respect to age, I refer to "physiological" age as opposed to "chronological" age. In other words, not how many years per se that you have lived on the planet, but at what age you are functioning and how many years you may be expected to live. Of two men who are chronologically 65 years old, one may be functioning like a 55-year-old and the other as an 80-year-old, and treatment needs to be tailored accordingly.

As surgery and radiation have competitive 15-year results and the demands and potential side effects of surgery are greater than that of radiation, at a certain age, radiotherapy becomes a prudent consideration.

Health status

If you are not in good health and do not have an expected ten-year life expectancy, there is usually no compelling reason to treat the prostate cancer as other health issues are likely to be of more concern than the prostate cancer.

In general, surgery should be reserved for healthy men who can tolerate an invasive surgical procedure and the general anesthesia necessary to undergo it. If your health is compromised, but you have a greater than ten-year life expectancy, radiation becomes a sensible management option.

Urinary symptoms

Benign prostate enlargement commonly accompanies aging, paralleling the increasing prevalence of prostate cancer with aging. As the prostate enlarges, it often—but not always—squeezes the urethral channel, making urination difficult and resulting in annoying symptoms and sleep disturbance. An enlarged prostate can act like a hand squeezing a garden hose, compromising the flow through the hose. The situation can be anything from a tolerable nuisance to one that has a huge impact on one's daily activities and quality of life.

The presence of Lower Urinary Tract Symptoms (LUTS) can be an important factor in guiding treatment options.

<u>Obstructive LUTS</u> consist of the following:

hesitancy—a stream that is slow to start

weak stream—a stream that lacks force

narrow stream—a thin stream

intermittency—a stream that starts and stops

straining—the need to use abdominal muscles to urinate

prolonged emptying time—excessive time to empty the bladder

incomplete emptying—inability to empty the bladder

<u>Irritative LUTS</u> consist of the following:

frequency—urinating more often than normal

nocturia—awakening from sleep to urinate

urgency—the sudden and strong desire to urinate

precipitancy—the need to get to the toilet in a hurry

urgency incontinence—the sudden and strong desire to urinate with the inability to get to the toilet in time to prevent leakage

The presence or absence of LUTS can be an important factor to help guide the most appropriate treatment options. For example, if a man diagnosed with prostate cancer has significant LUTS, a prostatectomy may be the best management option to treat both the cancer and the annoying symptoms, as opposed to radiation therapy that can worsen the LUTS.

Personal preferences

Our intention as urologists is not to dictate exactly what approach to take, as there are usually several competing management options, but to provide education, direction and guidance through the options, offering sensible and pragmatic advice based upon our knowledge and experience. Again, I truly believe in the FBSU test (Father, Brother, Son, Uncle test)— giving patients the same advice I would give to family members. Every man has different circumstances, priorities, medical issues, life expectancies and concerns about the side effects of treatment alternatives. Recognizing this, the opinions of the patient, family members and loved ones who have a clear understanding of the management options are of paramount importance in the ultimate choice of a treatment. The goal of this collaborative and shared decision-making process between patient and physician is to optimize medical decisions by helping patients choose the option they feel most comfortable with.

RISK CATEGORIZATION (This strategy is based upon the National Comprehensive Cancer Network guidelines)

Integrating the factors of tumor category, Gleason score, cancer volume, PSA, PSA density, supplemented with genomic testing, an individual case of prostate cancer can be assigned to one of five risk categories ranging from very low risk to very high risk. This risk categorization is helpful in predicting the future behavior of the prostate cancer and in the management decision-making process.

The following are the five risk groups and the criteria for membership in each:

Very Low Risk: T1-T2a; Gleason score 6; fewer than 3 cores with cancer; PTI less than 50% of cancer in each core; PSA < 10; PSA density < 0.15

Low Risk: T1-T2a; Gleason score 6; more than 3 cores with cancer; PTI greater than 50% of cancer in any core; PSA < 10

Intermediate Risk: T2b-T2c or Gleason score 7 or PSA 10-20

Within the intermediate risk category, further sub-stratification is as follows:

Favorable Intermediate Risk:

T1-T2a, Gleason score 6, PSA 10-20

T1-T2a, Gleason score 7 (3+4), PSA < 10

Unfavorable Intermediate Risk:

54

T2b, Gleason score 7 (3+4), PSA < 10

T1-T2, Gleason score 7 (3+4), PSA 10-20

T1-T2, Gleason score 7 (4+3), PSA < 20

High Risk: T3a or Gleason score 8-10 or PSA > 20

Very High Risk: T3b-T4 or Gleason grade 5 as the predominant grade (the first of the two Gleason grades in the Gleason score) or > 4 cores Gleason score 8-10

Chapter 14: How is Prostate Cancer Treated?

This chapter provides a brief overview of traditional treatment options based upon risk stratification. The chapters that follow will discuss each treatment option in detail.

It is important to understand that there is no one-size-fits-all treatment approach to prostate cancer as there are "competing" options, each with benefits that must be weighed against side effects. Many patients are fearful and confused about side effects that may occur after surgery or radiation—specifically, how frequently side effects occur, how severe they are, and how they are managed. Nowadays, side effects occur less frequently and are less severe than many imagine because of technical progress and advances in both the treatment of prostate cancer and in the management of side effects.

Treatment for cure is pursued when the prostate cancer is localized to the prostate, with the goal of eliminating all prostate cancer cells from the body. Localized cancer options are *robotic-assisted laparoscopic prostatectomy* and *prostate radiation therapy*. In general, if one is young and in good health, the option of choice is often surgical removal of the prostate as this is a highly effective means of long-term cure. Radiation therapy can be an excellent alternative to surgery with similar cure rates and less adverse effects and is often the option of choice in the older and less healthy population, as well as in men reluctant to undergo surgery.

Androgen deprivation therapy uses an injection of a medication to suppress levels of the male hormone testosterone to "castrate" levels, the same levels that would be achieved if the testes were surgically removed. *Active surveillance* is a means of vigilant tracking of the prostate cancer with no treatment per se aside from careful monitoring with plans for a change in strategy to active intervention if indicators worsen. *Observation* is a means of monitoring with the expectation of palliative therapy (relieving pain and alleviating other problems that may arise) if symptoms happen to develop or a change in exam or PSA suggests that symptoms are imminent.

Cryosurgery (freeze destruction of the prostate) and *high intensity focused ultrasound*, a.k.a. HIFU (heat destruction of the prostate) are alternative approaches, although less traditional than surgery or radiation therapy and are not listed in the treatment option outline that follows.

TREATMENT OPTIONS BASED UPON RISK STRATIFICATION

RALP (robotic-assisted laparoscopic prostatectomy)

RT (radiation therapy)

ADT (androgen deprivation therapy)

AS (active surveillance)

Observation

Very Low Risk

< 10-year life expectancy: observation

10-20-year life expectancy: AS

> 20-year life expectancy: AS or RALP or RT

Low Risk

< 10-year life expectancy: observation

> 10-year life expectancy: AS or RALP or RT

Certain factors increase the likelihood of progression on active surveillance and their presence may influence a low risk patient to pursue active treatment. These include the presence of perineural invasion on biopsy (cancer involving the space surrounding a nerve), African American race, family history of prostate cancer or a genetic predisposition to metastatic prostate cancer. Low risk men most likely will have localized disease and have a

90-95% recurrence-free survival rate 5 years after RALP or RT. Surgery and radiation in the low risk population generally do not improve survival before 10 years of follow-up as compared to active surveillance but reduce prostate cancer progression and the occurrence of metastases thereafter.

Intermediate Risk

< 10-year life expectancy: observation or RT + ADT 4-6 months

> 10-year life expectancy: RALP or RT + ADT 4-6 months

AS may be a possibility in selected patients with favorable intermediate risk prostate cancer, but this will incur a greater chance of developing metastases as compared with definitive treatment. Intermediate risk men have a 65-75% recurrence-free survival rate 5 years after RALP or RT. Patients with intermediate risk prostate cancer have improved survival when short-term ADT is combined with RT.

High Risk

RALP or RT + ADT 2-3 years

High risk prostate cancer is aggressive and incurs a likelihood of metastases and death. There is no place for AS, although observation is preferred in a man with a life expectancy of fewer than 5 years. Under the circumstances of symptomatic disease and limited life expectancy, ADT alone is a reasonable option. High risk men have 50% recurrence-free survival rate 5 years after RALP or RT. Combined modality therapy is likely to be needed, such as RT plus long-term ADT, or RALP plus adjuvant RT (radiotherapy given as soon as the healing process after RALP is completed).

Very High Risk

T3b-T4: RT + ADT 2-3 years or RALP (in select patients) or ADT alone

Lymph node spread: ADT or RT + ADT 2-3 years

Metastatic disease: ADT

Treatment for palliation of cancer is used when prostate cancer advances well beyond the confines of the prostate gland, often to the bony skeleton. In palliative therapy the goal is reduction in the severity of the symptoms resulting from the cancer, but not cure. ADT is most often used in this setting.

PSA FOLLOWING TREATMENT

No matter what the treatment, careful follow-up is imperative. Paramount is PSA—an excellent marker of the level of activity of prostate cancer. After successful RALP, the PSA should be undetectable; after successful radiation, the PSA should revert to a very low level and remain so.

After definitive treatment, a rising PSA may be the sole indication of the recurrence of prostate cancer, a condition known as biochemical recurrence. The important question that needs to be answered is whether the PSA elevation is due to local recurrence, systemic disease, or both, and how to distinguish the low risk from high risk patient.

A single abnormal PSA does not necessarily indicate that a biochemical failure has occurred. After RALP, biochemical failure becomes a consideration after the PSA is in the 0.2-0.4 range. In general, a low pre-treatment PSA, a lower grade, a lower stage, a longer time from definitive treatment to PSA relapse, and a longer PSA doubling time prognosticate a low likelihood for development of systemic metastases and a greater likelihood of local recurrence.

Salvage radiation therapy (RT following RALP, after a biochemical recurrence is noted) is an appropriate consideration for localized recurrence after RALP. Cryosurgery, HIFU, or ADT are considerations for biochemical failure due to localized recurrence after RT.

Military Metaphor: To combat and defeat prostate cancer, intelligence ("intel") will need to be gathered about the "enemy" and reconnaissance ("recon") missions will need to be deployed to survey and ascertain the strategic features of the enemy. Based upon intel and recon, many cases will require multimodal actions (different treatments that are combined). The multimodal approach can be thought of in terms of the different branches of the military that can work separately or in tandem to keep the enemy at bay. One can think of surgery as the Army with its ground forces using artillery and tactical weapons to mount a direct attack via the land, radiation therapy as the Air Force using gunfire on the enemy from the air and space, and androgen deprivation therapy (circulating through the blood) as the Naval Forces using the sea to their advantage. Chemotherapy, advanced hormonal therapy, immunotherapy and bone-targeted therapy in the event of prostate cancer progression can be thought of as Marines– specialty troops who can be deployed using to their advantage the latest and newest generation weapons in the event that the three main branches of the military fail to thwart the enemy.

Chapter 15: What is Active Surveillance (AS)?

"To do nothing, that's something."
—Samuel Shem, The House of God

The challenge for those treating prostate cancer is to predict the behavior of the cancer to best treat it appropriately—offering curative treatment to those with aggressive cancer but sparing the potential side effects of curative treatment in those who have non-aggressive cancer. The goal of active surveillance is to avoid treating cancers that do not have lethal or metastatic potential. Non-life-threatening, low risk prostate cancers are carefully monitored, avoiding active treatment or delaying it until there are signs of progression.

The ratio of lifetime likelihood of diagnosis of prostate cancer (about 1 in 9 men) to death from prostate cancer (about 1 in 40 men) points to the fact that many men with prostate cancer have an indolent (slow growing) cancer. On this basis, an alternative strategy to aggressive management of all men with prostate cancer is for careful follow-up, reserving curative intervention for if and when signs of progression develop.

Active surveillance involves rigorous monitoring and the willingness to have regular follow-ups. It is also appropriate for older men or those with serious health conditions.

Active surveillance was introduced in the mid-1990s and has gradually gained traction to the extent that this current time period can be thought of as the "era of active surveillance."

Eligibility criteria for active surveillance are the following (note that these are general guidelines and are modified in accordance with patient age, general health and other factors—certainly if one has a life expectancy of less than 10 years, he would be a good candidate for active surveillance):

- PSA less or equal to 10

- Gleason score 6, although active surveillance is occasionally used for low-volume Gleason 7 (3+4) cancer (Note that although some experts do not think that the term "cancer" is appropriate for Gleason 6 disease, recent studies have shown that a small percentage of men with Gleason 6 can potentially have local extension outside the prostate, supporting the argument for continuing to use the term cancer for these tumors.)

- Stage T1c-T2a

- Less than 3 cores with cancer

- Less than 50% of any one core involved

- Genomic testing confirming low risk for progression is an additional tool that can help guide eligibility

A general guide to the monitoring schedule is the following:

- PSA and DRE at least every 6 months

- Repeat biopsy ("confirmatory biopsy") one year following initial diagnosis, then periodically thereafter (I prefer annual biopsies for the first 3 years)

- Prostate MRI (not a substitute for repeat biopsy, but once serial biopsies have confirmed low risk cancer, can be used periodically in lieu of prostate biopsy)

Serial PSA levels are invaluable for men on active surveillance. PSA doubling time (PSADT)—the amount of time it takes for the PSA to double—is an excellent means of predicting prostate cancer behavior. A short PSA doubling time is usually indicative of an aggressive, rapidly growing tumor, whereas a long PSA doubling time is indicative of an indolent, slower growing tumor. A PSADT of less than 3 years is clearly associated with the potential for progression of prostate cancer.

The repeat biopsy is the most important component of the active surveillance protocol. There are three possible outcomes to follow-up biopsies: cancer-free, stable low risk cancer, and worsening cancer. A cancer-free pathology report is usually indicative of an excellent prognosis, insofar as the absence of cancer on repeated prostate biopsy (because the cancer is of such low volume) identifies men who are unlikely to have progressive prostate cancer. It does not mean that cancer is no longer present but implies that the cancer is extremely low volume and that the original biopsy discovered the "needle in the haystack." Stable low risk cancer is consistent with the original biopsy in terms of tumor volume and grade and indicates that the active surveillance protocol may be continued, sparing the patient the potential side effects of surgery, radiation or other modalities. Worsening cancer is demonstrated by a higher Gleason score or increased tumor volume as indicated by number of cores and percentage of tumor involvement per core. A higher Gleason score, increased tumor volume or a PSADT of less than 3 years will often result in a reclassification requiring a change in plan to active management with curative intent.

65-75% or so of men on active surveillance remain free of progression at five years, and definitive treatment is usually effective in the 25-35% who progress or elect active treatment for another reason.

Advantages of Active Surveillance:

• Avoids side effects and complications of immediate treatment

• Minimizes over-treatment of indolent prostate cancer

• Low cost

Disadvantages of Active Surveillance:

• Need for frequent and repeated testing and biopsies

• Anxiety of living with untreated prostate cancer

• Imprecise criteria for delayed intervention

• Delayed treatment may ultimately need to be more aggressive (with more potential side effects) compared to earlier intervention

• Delayed treatment may not be curative or as effective as earlier intervention

Chapter 16: What is Robotic-Assisted Laparoscopic Prostatectomy (RALP)?

Radical prostatectomy is the surgical removal of the entire prostate and the attached seminal vesicles. Upon excision, the detached urethra is sewn to the bladder neck to restore the continuity of the lower urinary tract. The goal is cancer control and preservation of urinary and sexual function. At the time of the prostatectomy, the pelvic lymph nodes are usually sampled, a consideration for any man undergoing RALP and a definite recommendation for those with unfavorable intermediate risk or high risk features. A pathologist microscopically examines the removed tissues and provides valuable information as to the precise pathological stage of the prostate cancer.

Before the availability of laparoscopy and robotics, prostatectomy was performed through large incisions—either retropubic (a lower abdominal incision) or perineal (an incision between the scrotum and anus)—with poorer visualization, more blood loss, less precision, more pain and longer hospital stays and recovery. With technical advances, the laparoscopic approach replaced the open technique, and more recently, the robot has further refined the laparoscopic approach.

ROBOTIC-ASSISTED LAPAROSCOPIC PROSTATECTOMY

With the advent of laparoscopy ("keyhole") surgery done via small portals and thereafter the development and refinement of surgical robotics, many advantages have accrued. Major surgical procedures are performed less invasively, with a reduction in blood loss, a brighter, sharper and magnified visual field for the surgeon, refined precision in the dissection of delicate tissue and facilitation of suturing. The urologist with a dedicated team of assistants harnesses the powers and advantages of robotic technology — an extraordinary example of human-machine symbiosis.

Initially, portals are placed via small incisions. As opposed to large incisions, these keyholes leave only small scars and cause limited pain. Through one of these portals, a camera is inserted to obtain an optically magnified, three-dimensional, high definition view of the surgical field. The camera can be manipulated, zoomed, rotated, etc. Robotic instruments that are mounted on the robot's arms are inserted through the portals. These include electric cautery (used to cut and coagulate tissue), scissors, forceps, scalpels, needle holders and other surgical tools.

In our practice, two board-certified urologic surgeons perform the surgery. One surgeon sits at a console remote from the patient and controls and maneuvers the robotic instruments while viewing the operation in real-time, while the other surgeon is positioned on the side of the patient and assists with instrument exchanges and aids in the dissection. An advantage of sitting at the console is that it is a comfortable, ergonomically favorable position that minimizes postural fatigue that often accompanies standing up for traditional open surgery. The surgeon's fingers are inserted into surgical joysticks that provide control of the instruments by using natural hand and wrist movements, with the system converting the surgeon's movements to precise, tremor-free robotic micro-movements. In addition to hand controls, the surgeon uses foot pedals to control the camera, focus, electrocautery and coagulation. Seven degrees of freedom (each direction a joint can move is a degree of freedom) are provided at the instrument tips. 540 degrees of pivoting (a full 360-degree rotation plus an additional 180-degree rotation) provide greater maneuverability than is possible with human hands or laparoscopic instruments.

RALP is currently the surgical approach of choice for removing a cancerous prostate gland due to the aforementioned refinements it provides in comparison to open and traditional laparoscopic surgery. Because of these advantages, in addition to less bleeding, less post-operative pain and shorter hospital stays, there are improved outcomes in terms of urinary control and sexual function as compared with the open approach.

RALP generally entails several hours under anesthesia and an overnight stay in the hospital. A catheter typically remains in the bladder for a week or so after the surgery. A unique benefit of RALP is that the removed tissue is available to be scrutinized in its entirety by the pathologist. The pathology report on the removed prostate, seminal vesicles, and lymph nodes provides important information regarding prognosis and helps determine if any other forms of therapy are indicated. If the report indicates that the cancer is all contained within the prostate capsule with normal margins, the prognosis is excellent. RALP is an excellent long-term means of cure of localized prostate cancer. Our goal as urologists is the "trifecta"—an undetectable PSA, excellent urinary control and satisfactory erections.

Adverse pathological features include the following:

- Perineural invasion or lympho-vascular invasion (growth of the cancer along the nerve, lymphatic or blood vessel branches)

- Extra-capsular extension (extension of the cancer beyond the prostate capsule)

- Positive surgical margins (cancer at the specimen edge)

- Seminal vesicle invasion (invasion into the seminal vesicles)

- Lymph node metastases (spread to the lymph nodes)

The neurovascular bundles (NVB)

The NVB are paired structures that provide nerve and blood supply to the penile erectile chambers, the prostate gland, the urethra, the rectum and the pelvic floor muscles (levator ani). The NVB are of particular importance with respect to sexual function since they contain the nerve control for initiating the erectile response as well as the emission and ejaculation of semen. The NVB are formed by branches of pelvic nerves that unite with blood vessels (both arteries and veins) that are contained within leaves of connective tissue. The NVB course down the sides of the prostate near the junction between the prostate and rectum.

Whenever possible, a nerve-sparing approach is performed to maximize the potential for erectile function and urinary control after the RALP. The challenge is that each NVB is quite delicate and has an intimate anatomic relation to the prostate and can easily be traumatized. If an area of cancer extension beyond the capsule is recognized at the time of RALP, all measures are taken to remove the cancer completely, often requiring incremental nerve sparing, tailored to the degree of cancer extension, which can range from partial nerve sparing to completely sacrificing the NVB.

For a young man with good sexual function and no medical co-morbidities who has a bilateral nerve sparing procedure, the ability to regain a penetrable erection one year following RALP will be in the 85-90% range with or without oral ED medications. These percentages will be less when only one side is spared. Excising the NVB on both sides will result in ED in virtually all men. It is important to know that the nerve-sparing approach does not absolutely guarantee the recovery of erections in all patients.

Advantages of RALP:

- A one-time procedure that intends to completely remove the cancerous organ and offers excellent long-term cancer control

- The pathology report on the removed prostate and sampled lymph nodes will offer staging and prognostic information

- Provides an excellent means of managing lower urinary tract symptoms due to benign prostate enlargement and prevents the future occurrence of symptomatic benign prostate enlargement, common in the aging male

- PSA should be undetectable after the procedure, so recurrences are easy to detect if PSA becomes detectable

- If RALP fails to cure the cancer, radiation therapy is available as a backup, potentially curative option

- The major complications, erectile dysfunction and urinary incontinence, are treatable

Disadvantages of RALP:

- A technically challenging, major operation that requires anesthesia, a hospital stay, a catheter and time lost from normal activities

- Potential over-treatment of low risk cancers

- Potential for adverse pathological findings that may require subsequent radiation therapy

- 20-25% will have a PSA recurrence, indicative of a limitation of surgery to cure the cancer in all cases

- Possibility of rectal injury, erectile dysfunction and urinary incontinence

- Dry ejaculation

- Possibility of penile shortening

- Possibility of bladder neck contracture—scar tissue where the bladder neck is sewn to the urethra, which may necessitate further procedures (but much less occurrence with robotic approach as opposed to open approach)

PSA after RALP

PSA after RALP should be undetectable. However, it is possible that prostate cancer cells had spread beyond the prostate before the prostatectomy, and at some point, these cells are capable of multiplying and producing a detectable PSA. If there is a PSA elevation following prostatectomy, it is usually an indication of a biochemical recurrence of the prostate cancer, although it can sometimes represent retained benign prostate tissue, in which case the PSA velocity should be expected to be very slow. The most widely accepted definition of a recurrence after radical prostatectomy is a PSA of 0.2 or higher, with a second confirmatory test to verify it. The most common site of recurrence after RALP is the prostate bed, the location where the prostate used to be.

Important factors governing the likelihood of prostate cancer progression after radical prostatectomy are the PSA doubling time (the longer the doubling time, the better the prognosis), the interval from surgery to the time of biochemical recurrence (the longer the interval, the better the prognosis) and the Gleason score (the lower the score, the better the prognosis). PSA doubling time less than 9 months, an interval to PSA recurrence of less than 3 years, and pathological Gleason score 8-10 are poor prognostic features suggesting microscopic metastatic disease.

"Adjuvant" radiation therapy is radiation therapy used after RALP for T3 disease, a means of significantly reducing the risk for PSA recurrence and metastasis and increasing survival. Alternatively, "salvage" radiation therapy is radiation therapy applied to the prostate bed after demonstration of a biochemical occurrence, an effective method to treat locally recurrent disease. Those with recurrent disease with poor prognostic features likely have both local and distant recurrences and are best treated with combined salvage radiation therapy and androgen deprivation therapy. Adjuvant or salvage radiation therapy can be highly effective, but may potentially exacerbate the side effects that occur after RALP.

Chapter 17: What is Radiation Therapy (RT)?

Radiation oncology is the medical specialty devoted to the use of radiation for the treatment of patients with cancer. Radiation therapy, a.k.a. radiotherapy, utilizes high-energy x-rays that kill prostate cancer cells by damaging their DNA. Radiation can be delivered externally (from a source outside of the body) or internally (from a source within the body). The former is known as external beam radiotherapy and the latter as brachytherapy. External radiotherapy, either alone or combined with brachytherapy, is a curative therapy for prostate cancer and is often used in combination with androgen deprivation therapy for patients with intermediate or high-risk disease.

EXTERNAL RADIATION THERAPY

The goal of external radiation therapy is to cure prostate cancer by delivering a precise dose of radiation to a defined target while minimizing the dose to the adjacent tissues. A machine called a linear accelerator generates and directs beams of x-rays to the prostate target. The daily dose is delivered five days a week over the course of 8-9 weeks to achieve a cumulative dose sufficient to kill the cancer cells. Each daily treatment is painless and is delivered in 10 minutes or so. An advantage of radiation therapy over surgery can be decreased side effects, with rare urinary incontinence and somewhat less erectile dysfunction.

External radiation therapy technology has undergone major refinements over the past few decades. Technology has evolved from conformal therapy that shaped the radiation beam to avoid adjacent structures, to intensity modulated radiotherapy (IMRT) that modulated the beam through various angles to further minimize the dose to adjacent organs, to the latest and most sophisticated technique—image guided radiation therapy (IGRT).

Image guided radiation therapy (IGRT) incorporates strategies to more accurately localize the prostate gland and optimize the radiation dose. Advances in radiotherapy imaging, planning and delivery systems have enabled unprecedented sophistication in the ability to target prostate cancer while sparing healthy tissue. Increasing the radiation dosage to the cancerous prostate gland has improved results and survival. Side effects are reduced because of less exposure to the bladder and rectum.

The prostate gland can move subtly in position from day to day, based upon the amount of urine in the bladder, gas and stool in the rectum and other factors. IGRT enables more precise localization of the exact position of the prostate, which reduces the radiation field. Without IGRT, the radiation field must be larger to account for the subtle changes in prostate size and movement, with the undesirable necessity for the radiation of healthy adjacent tissues. IGRT allows for fine adjustments in patient positioning to be made immediately before treatment, allowing reduced planning margins—the extra margin added to the clinical treatment volume because of uncertainties in prostate position due to prostate movement between radiotherapy treatments. Since the prostate location is precisely visualized using cone beam computerized tomography (CT) imaging, shifts in the treatment position can be made to correct for misalignment, reducing the planning margins and resulting in lower doses to adjacent tissues.

One such commonly used IGRT system is the Varian Rapid Arc system. After small gold markers (Visicoils) are implanted into the prostate gland, patients undergo CT simulation that creates 3-dimensional images of their anatomy, which allows conformal radiation planning. During the daily radiation treatment, a cone beam CT image of the prostate is obtained and by utilizing the Visicoils, fusion software allows accurate comparison of the daily prostate position to the planned position. Small shifts in the treatment position are made to correct for prostate movement, eliminating the need for wider radiotherapy margins that would expose more healthy tissues to the radiation dose. RapidArc is a volumetric arc therapy that delivers a precisely sculpted 3-dimensional dose distribution with a single 360-degree rotation. Since RapidArc delivers treatments two to eight times faster than other systems, it is more precise and more convenient for the patient.

Aside from definitive treatment of prostate cancer, additional uses of external radiation are for adjuvant, salvage and palliative purposes:

Adjuvant radiation therapy

External radiation can be used as adjuvant therapy after prostatectomy when the pathology report demonstrates unfavorable features that incur a high risk of recurrence, including: invasion of the prostate capsule, cancer at the surgical margin, seminal vesicle invasion and/or lymph node involvement. Radiotherapy is delivered to the bed of the prostate to "sterilize" the remaining cancer cells to prevent progression and metastases.

Salvage radiation therapy

External radiation can be used as salvage therapy for those patients who develop biochemical recurrence, defined as a PSA elevation after surgery. In salvage radiation therapy, radiotherapy is delivered to the bed of the prostate to "sterilize" the remaining cancer cells to prevent progression and metastases.

Palliative radiation therapy

In addition to curative efforts, external radiation is used as palliative therapy to eliminate pain and improve skeletal integrity for those with metastatic disease to the bones. 75% or so of patients with painful bony metastases will have pain relief after palliative radiation is administered to the sites of concern.

Cyberknife is a technology originally conceived for treating brain and spinal tumors that has been adapted for prostate cancer. Also known as stereotactic radiotherapy, it is a form of high intensity focused radiation that can be completed over a course of 5 sessions as opposed to 44 sessions of standard radiotherapy and is thus also known as hypo-fractionated radiotherapy. Its proponents claim that it is more "surgical" than standard radiotherapy, with reduced radiation dosing to adjacent organs. A computer-controlled robotic arm swivels to shoot dozens of radiation beams from many angles, resulting in high doses that are "sculpted" to the cancer. Although the concept of an accelerated and compressed course of radiation is convenient and inviting, data on the long-term effectiveness and urinary and bowel consequences of the Cyberknife are not yet available.

Proton beam therapy uses heavy particle beams (protons) generated by linear accelerators or cyclotrons as opposed to standard radiotherapy (that uses photons). These beams are difficult to produce and control, but possess a unique physical characteristic called the "Bragg peak" that allows for a sharp edge that can reduce the dose to tissue lying a few millimeters from the intended target. Proton therapy is excellent for tumors that are close to the surface and for tumors of the brain and spine but its long-term effectiveness for prostate cancer remains unknown. There is an increasing interest in this modality, but proton therapy remains a contentious issue in the field of radiation oncology.

Radiation therapy survival rates

Radiation therapy and RALP have similar 15-year survival rates with results being best for low risk disease and less effective for intermediate and high risk cancers. Serum PSA is widely accepted as the best marker for monitoring the effectiveness of treatment. Unlike surgery, patients successfully treated with radiation therapy still have a prostate gland and are not expected to achieve an undetectable PSA. An acceptable PSA following radiation is a low PSA (<1.0 ng/ml), which typically reaches its lowest point (nadir) 18-24 months after completion of therapy.

It is possible for prostate cancer cells to have spread beyond the prostate before radiation therapy, and at some point, these cells are capable of multiplying and producing a detectable PSA. Biochemical failure is defined as 3 consecutive PSA rises over several months. In general, the shorter the PSA doubling time, the worse the prognosis. Another definition of biochemical failure is a PSA rise of 2.0 above the lowest point. Serial PSA testing is particularly important after radiation therapy since it is possible for the PSA to "bounce" (a.k.a. "spike" or "bump") up temporarily only to return to normal levels thereafter. This bounce phenomenon occurs most commonly with brachytherapy and usually within the first two years following the radiation. Although the precise cause is unknown, it is theorized to be a delayed inflammatory reaction to the radiation therapy.

Radiation side effects

Radiation toxicity is divided into acute and chronic. Acute toxicity develops during the treatment period and may consist of fatigue and/or urinary frequency and irritation due to inflammation of the urethra (the channel that drains the bladder). Less commonly, patients develop frequent loose bowel movements due to irritation of the rectum. Chronic toxicity develops beyond 3 months or more after completing radiation therapy. Injury to the microvasculature (small blood vessels) of the organs adjacent to the prostate can cause proctitis, with intermittent rectal bleeding in 10% of patients and cystitis, with intermittent urinary tract bleeding in a small percentage of men. Erectile dysfunction occurs in 30-40% of men, which often responds to oral erectile dysfunction medications.

Fact: In the early phase, radiation induces inflammation and edema (tissue swelling) of the prostate whereas in the late phase it induces microvascular damage (damage to the smallest blood vessels), tissue hypoxemia (low concentrations of oxygen) and fibrosis (scarring).

An absorbable hydrogel spacer is a new means of providing protection to the rectum in men who opt to undergo radiation therapy for prostate cancer. The anatomic proximity of the rectum and the prostate puts the rectum at risk for radiation exposure and toxicity. This absorbable material is implanted via an injection in the perineum (area between the scrotum and the anus) into the space between the prostate and rectum. The creation of increased space between the rectum and prostate results in a reduced radiation dose to the rectum, which diminishes rectal pain and decreases long-term rectal, urinary and sexual complications. The absorbable hydrogel spacer lasts over the course of the radiation therapy and thereafter is gradually resorbed by the body. The only prostate cancer spacing device that is approved by the FDA for use in the USA is SpaceOAR, which uses polyethylene glycol as the spacing material.

Advantages of external radiotherapy:

- Excellent cancer control without major invasive surgery and anesthesia

- Can treat locally-advanced cancer that extends beyond the prostate

- Outpatient

- Less urinary control side effects than surgery

- Can be used for men who have had prior prostate surgery and a local recurrence

Disadvantages of external radiotherapy:

- Need for multiple treatment visits to the radiation center

- Technically-challenging procedure requiring sophisticated equipment and multidisciplinary interactions among radiation oncologists, radiologists, medical physicists and computer planners

- Leaves prostate intact in the body (as opposed to completely removing the diseased organ)

- Short-term side effects include fatigue, urinary frequency and frequent bowel movements

- Long-term side effects include the possibility of bladder bleeding and irritative lower urinary tract symptoms (radiation cystitis), rectal bleeding and irritative bowel symptoms (radiation proctitis) and erectile dysfunction

- If radiation fails, "salvage" prostatectomy is possible but it is a much more challenging surgery with more significant side effects because of scarring around the prostate gland; other options for radiation failure are androgen deprivation therapy, cryosurgery and high intensity focused ultrasound

- Small increase in secondary cancers including those of the bladder and rectum

PROSTATE BRACHYTHERAPY

Brachytherapy is a minimally invasive procedure in which radioactive sources are implanted directly within the prostate gland.

Low dose rate brachytherapy (LDR) uses titanium-encapsulated radioactive seeds (each about the size of a grain of rice) that are implanted directly into the prostate. After the radiation is "spent," the seeds that remain are harmless "shells." LDR brachytherapy is largely of historical interest since it is rarely used anymore.

High dose rate brachytherapy (HDR) uses temporary flexible plastic needles that are placed through the perineum and are used as a vehicle through which Iridium–192 wires are advanced into the prostate gland. A computer-controlled system calculates how long the "hot" wires stay in each dwell position within the needles, which determines the delivered dose. Once each treatment is finished, the radioactive wires are removed from the prostate. Three fractions of high dose rate brachytherapy are delivered over a course of a 24-hour hospital stay. HDR is typically reserved for those patients with high risk disease—Gleason scores 8-10, increased tumor volume and elevated PSA. It is most often done in conjunction with long-term androgen deprivation therapy.

Advantages of HDR brachytherapy:

- Delivery of a high dose of radiation into prostate with minimal radiation to healthy adjacent tissues

- Short hospitalization and rapid recovery

- Ability to treat high risk prostate cancer

Disadvantages of HDR brachytherapy:

- Need for anesthesia

- Need for urinary catheter

- Short-term discomfort and blood in the urine from plastic needles sutured into perineal area

Chapter 18: What is Androgen Deprivation Therapy (ADT)?

ANDROGEN DEPRIVATION THERAPY (ADT)

"Androgen" refers to male sex hormones, the main one of which is testosterone. Androgen deprivation therapy (ADT), a.k.a. hormonal therapy, is a means of managing prostate cancer by reducing levels of testosterone. Testosterone—90-95% of which is produced in the testicles—stimulates both benign and malignant prostate growth and its suppression with ADT restrains this growth.

For years, ADT has been the standard of care for advanced prostate cancer. Although it does not cure prostate cancer, lowering testosterone levels often makes prostate cancers shrink and grow more slowly and many patients will experience long-term remissions. Although it delays disease progression, the effects on survival are less clear. Because of side effects, ADT should only be used when clearly indicated and avoided when possible.

It is important to know that given enough time, prostate cancer cells are capable of mutating and ultimately becoming able to thrive in a low testosterone environment, a condition referred to as castrate resistant prostate cancer (CRPC).

ADT is useful in the following circumstances:

- As a delaying tactic because of the need to defer treatment

- In a man who desires treatment, but is unable to tolerate surgery or radiation because of poor health or advanced age

- In conjunction with radiation therapy since radiation and ADT have a synergistic effect (combined effect is greater than sum of separate effects)

- Prior to surgery, radiation, or ablative therapies to shrink the prostate

- To treat surgery or radiation failures

- As primary treatment for metastatic disease

ADT for prostate cancer can be achieved either surgically or medically:

Orchiectomy (surgical castration) is an operation in which the urologist removes the testicles. With the source of testosterone removed, most prostate cancers stop growing or shrink for a time. This is a simple outpatient procedure and is the least expensive and most uncomplicated way to reduce testosterone levels in the body. Unlike other methods of lowering testosterone levels, it is permanent and irreversible, and many men—understandably so—do not relish the concept of having their testicles removed. However, it is a possible choice for someone who favors an inexpensive and one-and-done approach to ADT.

Luteinizing hormone-releasing hormone (LHRH) analogs (also called LHRH agonists) lower testosterone levels as effectively as surgical castration, only chemically as opposed to surgically. They are the most commonly used means of ADT in the United States. LHRH analogs are given by needle injection either monthly or every 3, 4, or 6 months. The LHRH analogs available in the United States include leuprolide (Lupron, Viadur, Eligard), goserelin (Zoladex), and triptorelin (Trelstar).

When LHRH analogs are initially given, testosterone production increases before it falls to very low levels. This effect is called the "flare" or "surge" phenomenon. Men whose cancer has spread to the bones may experience bone pain because of this initial surge in testosterone. If the cancer has spread to the spine, even a short-term increase in cancer growth could compress the spinal cord and cause pain or paralysis. This flare can be avoided by giving anti-androgen medications for a few weeks before starting treatment with LHRH analogs or, alternatively, using a luteinizing hormone-releasing hormone antagonist.

Luteinizing hormone-releasing hormone (LHRH) antagonists are a newer class of medication that reduce testosterone without the flare. Degarelix (Firmagon) is an LHRH antagonist that induces "castrate" levels of testosterone within 3 days of the injection.

Possible side effects of all forms of ADT may include the following:

• hot flashes

• diminished sex drive

• erectile dysfunction

• breast tenderness and growth of breast tissue

• osteoporosis (bone thinning), which can lead to broken bones

• anemia (low red blood cell count)

• decreased mental acuity

• loss of muscle mass

• increase in body fat

• weight gain

• fatigue

• weakness

• altered lipid profiles: increase in cholesterol, triglycerides, and decrease in HDL ("good") cholesterol

• increased insulin resistance, type 2 diabetes and coronary disease

• depression

Anti-androgens block the body's ability to use testosterone, thus "starving" prostate cancer cells from being stimulated by testosterone. Their premise for being used is that even with LHRH analogs, LHRH antagonists or following surgical removal of the testes, small amounts of testosterone made by the adrenal glands can stimulate prostate cancer growth. Anti-androgen treatment may be combined with LHRH analogs, antagonists or surgical castration as first-line hormone therapy. This is called "combined androgen blockade" and functions to block adrenal as well as testicular testosterone. There is still some debate as to whether combined androgen blockade is more effective than using LHRH analog, LHRH antagonist or surgical castration alone.

First generation anti-androgens include bicalutamide (Casodex), flutamide (Eulexin), and nilutamide (Nilandron). Ketoconazole (Nizoral), although primarily used to treat fungal infections, can also be used as second-line hormonal therapy to treat advanced prostate cancer, although concerns about side effects encouraged the development of newer-generation anti-androgens, including enzalutamide (Xtandi), abiraterone (Zytiga), and apalutamide (Erleada). Side effects of anti-androgens in patients already treated with LHRH agonists, LHRH antagonists or surgical castration are usually not serious. Diarrhea is the major side effect, although seizures, nausea, liver problems, and fatigue can also occur. Anti-androgens are commonly added to LHRH analogs, LHRH antagonists or surgical castration when the latter are no longer working effectively, as reflected by a rise in PSA.

Controversies in ADT

There are many ADT issues that lack a clear consensus.

<u>Early vs. delayed treatment</u>

Some urologists feel that ADT works better if it is started as soon as possible after the diagnosis of advanced stage prostate cancer has been made, even if the patient is feeling well. These circumstances include the following: high stage (T3), high Gleason score, metastases to lymph nodes, and/or if the PSA starts rising after initial therapy. Alternatively, other urologists feel that because of side effects and the probability that the cancer could become resistant to ADT therapy sooner, treatment should not be started until after symptoms appear.

<u>Intermittent vs. continuous hormone therapy</u>

Since many prostate cancers treated with ADT become resistant after several years, some urologists advise intermittent (on-again, off-again) cycles of treatment. ADT is stopped once the PSA level drops to a low level and when the PSA level begins to rise, the ADT is re-started. An advantage of intermittent treatment is minimizing side effects of ADT, with the return of testosterone to near normal levels fostering better sexual function and less ADT side effects.

Reducing risk of ADT complications

Since ADT can have negative effects including fatigue and loss in muscle and bone mass, it is important to take measures to minimize these potential complications. Studies have clearly demonstrated that physical exercise, including aerobic and resistance training, will help maintain muscle and bone mass and improve fatigue and vitality. More about this in the chapter on bone health.

Chapter 19: What are Focal Ablative Therapies?

Focal ablative therapies are means of using energy—heating, freezing, etc.—to target and destroy defined portions of the prostate gland that contain "clinically significant" cancer. The use of focal ablative therapies requires precise imaging and pathological mapping of the prostate cancer, facilitated by the increasing popularity of MRI-guided biopsies. Focal ablation is best considered for low risk or low-volume intermediate risk cancer, whereas whole gland treatment is better for high risk or high-volume intermediate risk prostate cancer. Optimal candidates for focal therapy have a single MRI detectable lesion that correlates with pathological T1c-T2a Gleason 3+3 or 3+4 cancer, PSA less than 15, and a life expectancy exceeding 10 years.

"Focal" refers to treating only the region of concern, sparing the remainder of the prostate. "Ablative" refers to the destruction of tissue. The challenge is that prostate cancer is often multifocal, with disease present in multiple areas and involving both sides of the prostate. Focal therapies are based on the theory that although prostate cancer is usually multifocal, there is often a single "index" area that contains the most aggressive, at-risk disease, which is the region that is targeted. Quality imaging and mapping biopsies of the prostate are essential in order to determine the precise location of the index area. A problem with MRI is that it can underestimate the size of the index area and can miss some clinically significant cancers. Focal therapies, although theoretically advantageous in sparing portions of the prostate, pose the risk of leaving cancer untreated. Focal ablation can potentially serve as a "bridging" therapy between the extremes of active surveillance and active treatment (surgery or radiotherapy).

When ablative therapies are used to treat the entire prostate gland, significant side effects are often incurred. These include a prolonged need for a catheter, bothersome lower urinary tract symptoms, sloughing (passage of dead tissue through the urethra), urethral scarring and sexual issues. These side effects are less of a concern when ablative therapy is directed focally at only the region of concern.

Cryosurgery, a.k.a. cryotherapy or cryoablation, freezes prostate cancer cells. Prostate "frostbite" disrupts the cell membranes and the blood supply of prostate cancer cells, resulting in the destruction of the frozen tissue. As it is challenging to achieve uniform cold temperatures throughout larger prostate glands, prostate size is an important factor in selecting patients who are appropriate for this means of treatment. Cryosurgery incurs a very high risk of erectile dysfunction.

Freezing is achieved using cryoprobes that are positioned strategically within the prostate gland (similarly to how needles are placed into the prostate for brachytherapy radiation) using ultrasound guidance via a probe placed in the rectum and a perineal template. Pressurized argon gas is the medium used to freeze tissue. The procedure is performed under anesthesia with legs up in stirrups. To avoid damaging the urethra, it is warmed with a warming catheter that uses helium gas. Devices called thermocouples precisely monitor temperatures. A tissue temperature of –40 to –50 degrees Centigrade is achieved. Under most circumstances, the prostate is subjected to two cycles of freezing and thawing. The procedure can usually be done on an outpatient basis, with the patient sent home with a catheter for 1-3 weeks.

"Primary" cryosurgery is most effective for men with localized low and intermediate risk prostate cancer who are not suitable candidates for prostatectomy or radiation therapy and are not sexually functional nor interested in being sexually active. If the prostate is large, androgen deprivation therapy is useful to reduce the prostate volume and allow for more effective results. Freezing extending beyond the capsule of the prostate can potentially treat extra-capsular disease. "Salvage" cryosurgery is used for recurrent prostate cancer following radiation therapy.

Cryosurgery is still considered by many to be an emerging therapy and not quite in the same league as prostatectomy and radiotherapy. However, technological improvements in hardware and software have substantially improved the current generation of cryosurgery as compared to previous iterations.

Advantages of Cryosurgery:

• Outpatient procedure with minimal time lost from normal activities

• Relatively non-invasive

• Can be repeated if necessary

• Can target prostate cancer while sparing uninvolved areas of the prostate

Disadvantages of Cryosurgery:

• Attempted targeted treatment of cancer may unknowingly leave behind cancerous prostate tissue

• Need for prolonged bladder catheterization

• Potential damage to the urethra and rectum resulting in a recto-urethral fistula, an abnormal connection between these two structures, especially after salvage cryosurgery

• Urethral sloughing (passage of dead tissue through the urethra) resulting in urethral scarring and urinary difficulties, which occurs more commonly in men who have had previous procedures for benign prostate enlargement

• Pelvic pain (usually short term)

• Urinary issues including obstructive and irritative lower urinary tract symptoms and incontinence

• Erectile dysfunction is an expected outcome

• Rare pubic bone osteomyelitis (bone infection), especially after salvage cryosurgery

High-intensity focused ultrasound (HIFU) is a minimally invasive, alternative means of treating localized prostate cancer using thermal energy. It was approved by the FDA in 2015, although it has been available since 1995. Over the years, there have been numerous advances in both the HIFU software and hardware. Currently there are two main systems in use in the United States, the Ablatherm and the Sonablate.

Under anesthesia, a probe that generates high-intensity ultrasound waves is placed in the rectum. HIFU waves are delivered to the target area within the prostate to destroy cancer cells by means of heat destruction, without damaging tissue in the ultrasound beam pathway. A rectal cooling system is utilized to protect the rectum.

Overlapping target areas are defined and treated over the course of the 1-4 hours that it takes to do the procedure. Similar to cryosurgery, HIFU can be used either as "primary" therapy or alternatively as "salvage" therapy for recurrent prostate cancer following radiation failure. It can be used focally, to ablate half the prostate or to ablate the total prostate gland.

In addition to the thermal effect (heating tissue up to 85 degrees Centigrade), HIFU also functions via a mechanical effect (prostate cancer cell wall rupture) and a tissue effect (prostate cancer cell death and scarring).

If necessary, trans-urethral resection of the prostate (a procedure to create a channel through the prostate gland), is performed prior to HIFU to reduce the size of the prostate and minimize the possibility of urinary difficulties after the procedure, since urinary obstruction due to scarring and prostatic tissue sloughing are the most common side effects. A catheter is generally required for 3-7 days following the procedure.

Numerous long-term studies with over 10-year follow-up from Europe have shown cancer-free status equivalent to surgery or radiation. Since FDA approval, HIFU is considered by many as an attractive procedure, especially for less aggressive, relatively favorable or low volume disease. HIFU provides a better chance of preserving sexual function as compared to surgery or cryotherapy. A major challenge is the fact that many insurance companies do not yet pay for HIFU. At the current time, Medicare covers the HIFU facility fee, but not the professional fee. Most commercial insurances do not cover HIFU, although some cover salvage HIFU and some provide coverage on a case-to-case basis.

Advantages of HIFU:

- Outpatient, non-invasive procedure with little time lost from normal activities

- Minimal side effects, especially with targeted therapy

- Can be repeated if necessary

- Can target prostate cancer while sparing uninvolved areas of the prostate

- Better odds at preserving erections

Disadvantages of HIFU:

- Difficulty in treating the entire prostate when prostate is very large (although second generation device has a much greater reach)

- Attempted targeted treatment of cancer may unknowingly leave behind cancerous prostate tissue

- Requirement for general anesthesia

- Heat damage of nerves causing erectile dysfunction in approximately 30% of patients undergoing full gland treatment

- Rare recto-urethral fistula, especially after salvage HIFU

- Rare pubic bone osteomyelitis (bone infection), especially after salvage HIFU

Additional focal therapies under investigation

As of now, these forms of focal ablation are investigational and experimental. Clinical trials are limited by short-term follow up and it will take a number of years to accrue the data necessary to gauge their success.

MRI-guided focal laser ablation uses MRI to image and identify the cancerous region of concern. A laser fiber is guided into the interior of this selected region and laser energy is used to focally destroy it.

Irreversible electroporation uses pulsed, low-energy direct current to create micropores in cell membranes that lead to their rupture and destruction.

<u>Vascular targeted photodynamic therapy</u> ablates the tissue of concern via trans-perineal or trans-rectal laser activation of an intravenously given vascular photosensitizer. By exposure to a certain wavelength of light, the light-activated photosensitizer produces free radicals that cause the focal ablation.

Focal ablative therapies are emerging options that show promise in terms of short-term cancer results and a relatively favorable side effect profile, but they require further evaluation, clinical trials and follow up to assess their long-term cancer outcomes.

Chapter 20: What is Castration-Resistant Prostate Cancer (CRPC)?

Not all primary treatments for prostate cancer are curative, which can result in recurrent cancer. Many patients with such a recurrence will be cured or sustain a remission with a secondary treatment, e.g., radiation therapy following radical prostatectomy or androgen deprivation therapy following radiation therapy.

Those who will eventually die of prostate cancer progress through a sequence of discrete progressive stages including: "biochemical recurrence" (PSA rises after treatment) to "non-metastatic castration-sensitive prostate cancer" (PSA declines in response to androgen deprivation therapy) to "non-metastatic castration-resistant prostate cancer" (PSA rises despite androgen deprivation therapy) to "metastatic castration-resistant prostate cancer."

Biochemical recurrence following primary treatment

20-25% of men after prostatectomy will experience a biochemical recurrence within 10 years of surgery, despite the surgery performed by the most proficient and talented urological surgeons. This often responds to radiation therapy, although a percentage of patients will have an initial satisfactory response to the radiation (PSA drops to undetectable levels), but subsequently experience a second biochemical recurrence, indicative of a failure of the radiation therapy to cure the recurrence. Similarly, a small percentage of men after primary radiation therapy will experience a biochemical recurrence, despite the therapy delivered by highly competent radiation oncologists.

Biochemical recurrences are typically due to "micro-metastases," small numbers of cancer cells that spread from the primary tumor site to a separate part of the body and are undetectable despite the use of the most advanced imaging methods available. These cells can remain dormant for years and are the reason behind the importance for long-term follow up of any patient who has been treated for prostate cancer.

CASTRATE-RESISTANT PROSTATE CANCER (CRPC)

When biochemical recurrence occurs after surgery, radiation or adjuvant or salvage radiation following surgery, androgen deprivation therapy (ADT) is commonly started. Even after surgery followed by radiation eventually followed by ADT with the achievement of castrate levels of testosterone (blood levels < 50 ng/dl), 10-20% of patients will develop resistance to ADT within 5 years, manifested with a rising PSA or imaging evidence of prostate cancer progression. This is castration resistant prostate cancer (CRPC). Historically, CRPC was also referred to as "hormone-resistant prostate cancer" or "hormone-refractory prostate cancer." The average time to the occurrence of CRPC after starting ADT is 19 months. 30-40% of men with non-metastatic CRPC will progress to metastatic CRPC within 18-24 months.

The longer the exposure a patient has had to ADT, the more likely the prostate cancer cells can adapt, mutate and develop unique ways to protect themselves throughout the course of therapy, resulting in the prostate cancer cells thriving, growing, and spreading. Mutations can even result in the prostate cancer cells producing their own testosterone. The ability of a prostate cancer cell to survive and thrive varies from individual to individual and is influenced by genetics, environmental exposures, medications used to treat the prostate cancer, and an individual's immune system. Regardless of whether the CRPC is metastatic or not, all patients with CRPC are advised to continue with ADT to maintain castrate levels of testosterone, since testosterone is often a primary driver of the cancer. The good news is that in patients with metastatic CRPC, numerous new options are available that will be reviewed in detail in the pages that follow.

When prostate cancer progresses despite ADT, it can be asymptomatic and noted only because of a rising PSA, or it can be symptomatic, most commonly causing pain from bone metastases. The initial approach is to ensure that castrate levels of testosterone have been achieved. When a patient is diagnosed with CRPC, it is important to obtain staging information via imaging studies that may include computerized tomography, bone scan and perhaps some of the advanced imaging techniques discussed in the chapter that follows. After imaging is complete, a patient can be classified as not having metastatic spread (M0) or having metastatic spread (M1).

Genetic testing in men with CRPC

More than 20% of men with metastatic CRPC have defects in those genes that repair DNA, including BRCA, ATM, MMR, etc. Men with metastatic CRPC should have genetic testing and DNA sequencing of the cancer, or at a minimum have the tumor tested for certain biomarkers and assessment of genetic mutations.

Defective DNA repair genes may predict the response to PARP (poly-ADP-ribose polymerase) inhibitors that repair damaged DNA, currently undergoing clinical trials, as well as platinum-based chemotherapy. 5-10% of prostate cancers have MMR mutations and MSI (microsatellite instability—the condition that results from the MMR mutation) and may be candidates for immune checkpoint inhibitors.

Anti-androgens

Anti-androgens are medications that function to block the action of testosterone or compete with the binding of testosterone at the cellular level, resulting in the testosterone rendered incapable of stimulating the growth of the prostate cancer cell.

In the case of non-metastatic CRPC, if an anti-androgen has not been used, it is worthwhile to trial a medication of this class in addition to the LHRH analog or LHRH antagonist. First generation anti-androgens include bicalutamide (Casodex), flutamide (Eulexin) and nilutamide (Nilandron). Ketoconazole (Nizoral), although primarily used to treat fungal infections, is also used as second-line hormonal therapy to treat advanced prostate cancer via suppression of adrenal testosterone synthesis, although concerns about side effects have encouraged the development of the newest-generation agents.

New options to manage CRPC

Years ago, once CRPC occurred, the only option was chemotherapy with do-cetaxel. However, since 2010, there have been unparalleled changes in the field of advanced prostate cancer with the availability of numerous new-generation treatments capable of improving the quality of life and survival for those with CRPC. Pharmaceutical companies have created the following complex and memorable names for some of the novel medications: cabazi-taxel (Jevtana), denosumab (Xgeva), enzalutamide (Xtandi) abiraterone (Zytiga), and radium 223 (Xofigo). The newest entry is apalutamide (Erlea-da), FDA approved in 2018 for non-metastatic CRPC. These new treatments can be sub-categorized into advanced hormonal therapy, bone-targeted therapy, immunotherapy, and cytotoxic therapy.

Fact: Most of the brand names of these new agents have 5-7 letters, 3 syllables, begin with rare consonants and end in a vowel. If they could be used in a game of Scrabble, they would be of great value!

Advanced hormonal therapy

Abiraterone (Zytiga), approved by the FDA in 2011, works by inhibiting an enzyme in the adrenal steroid biosynthesis pathway, which blocks the pro-duction of testosterone and other testosterone-like hormones. Recall that one of the mechanisms of resistance to ADT is the ability of the prostate cancer cells to produce their own testosterone; Zytiga can prevent this from occurring. It must be used in conjunction with steroids to counteract side effects including high blood pressure, electrolyte abnormalities and fatigue.

A recently published clinical trial in 2018 demonstrated that the addition of Zytiga and prednisone to ADT significantly increased overall survival and decreased the risk of prostate cancer progression in men with newly diag-nosed metastatic castrate-sensitive prostate cancer, leading to a new FDA approval in 2018.

Enzalutamide (Xtandi), FDA approved in 2012, is a second-generation anti-androgen that works by blocking the activation of the androgen receptor by testosterone. In order for testosterone to function, it must first bind to the androgen receptor to activate it, after which it gets transported into the nu-cleus of the cell. Xtandi offers an advantage over the first-generation anti-androgens in that it binds with a stronger affinity to the androgen receptor.

It was originally approved only for metastatic CRPC, but because studies showed that it delayed metastases and offered a survival benefit to men with non-metastatic CRPC, it was FDA approved in July 2018 for use in men with non-metastatic CRPC. Potential side effects include fatigue, back pain, diarrhea, constipation, joint aches, cardiac adverse effects, high blood pressure, increased liver enzymes and, rarely, seizures.

Apalutamide (Erleada) in 2018 became the first FDA approved treatment for non-metastatic CRPC. Erleada works by blocking the activation of the androgen receptor by testosterone, with similar properties to enzalutamide, bicalutamide, and nilutamide. Clinical studies have demonstrated its ability to significantly delay the time to symptomatic progression, metastasis and death. Side effects include rash, hypothyroidism, fractures, and rare seizures.

Bone-targeted therapy

Bone metastases are the first site of metastases in the majority of patients with prostate cancer. Prostate cancer cells taking residence in bones can disrupt bone health and cause pain, pathological fractures and compression of nerves and the spinal cord in the circumstance of vertebral metastases. The combination of an aging male, prostate cancer bone metastases and the use of androgen deprivation therapy (which further accelerates bone loss) creates the perfect storm for the aforementioned bone maladies, referred to as "skeletal related events" (SRE). SRE include pathological fractures, spinal cord compression, and bone pain or impending fracture requiring the necessity for radiation therapy or surgery.

Fact: The condition of prostate cancer that has spread to the bones is referred to as "metastatic prostate cancer" as distinguished from "primary bone cancer."

Fortunately, medications are available that help fortify bones that have been weakened either by the accelerated bone loss from androgen deprivation therapy or from the presence of the cancer cells within the bones. Bone "anti-resorptive therapy" helps strengthen bones by driving calcium into the bones, decreasing the risk of SRE by reducing the amount of bone broken down by the body.

Zoledronic acid (Zometa) is a bisphosphonate given as a 15-minute infusion that is used to prevent SRE and to alleviate bone pain from metastatic CRPC. It is now infrequently used because clinical trials have demonstrated that Xgeva is better than Zometa in delaying or preventing SRE and does not impair kidney function as Zometa can.

Denosumab (Prolia) is used for patients on ADT (who have not yet developed bone metastases) to help maintain bone health and limit bone loss, used as 60 mg injection every six months.

Denosumab (Xgeva) is used for patients with a rising PSA despite ADT and for patients with bone metastases, used as 120 mg injection every four weeks.

A dental exam is recommended before initiation of the aforementioned bone-targeted therapies because of the potential side effect of osteonecrosis (death of bone tissue from lack of blood supply) of the jaw, a rare complication. Routine dental checkups every 6 months are advised.

Xofigo (Radium 223 Dichloride) is a radiopharmaceutical drug approved by the FDA in 2013 to treat CRPC metastatic to the bones. One injection is given intravenously every 4 weeks for a total of 6 doses. It is prescribed for patients with minimally symptomatic or symptomatic bone metastatic CRPC requiring analgesic medication, who have no lymph node enlargement greater than 3 cm in diameter and have no spread of the prostate cancer to organs including the lungs, liver, etc.

Xofigo mimics calcium and forms complexes at areas of increased bone turnover. It contains the radioactive material radium 223, which works at the site of bone metastases, emitting radiation that has an anti-cancer effect by inducing breaks in tumor cell DNA and causing cell death. It can be absorbed by other organs, particularly those that are very active, including bone marrow (where blood cells are produced) and the digestive system, which can result in side effects in those tissues. Anemia, low white blood cell counts, low platelet counts as well as bone pain, nausea, vomiting, diarrhea and swelling of the arms and legs may occur. Despite potential side effects, Xofigo has been a valuable addition to the CRPC treatment resources because it delays the time to symptomatic bone metastases and symptomatic SRE, reduces bone cancer pain, and provides a survival benefit. Furthermore, it has less bone marrow toxicity compared to the previous generation radiopharmaceuticals.

Immunotherapy

The immune system is the body's natural defense against infection and cancer. In patients with advancing prostate cancer, the immune system is often neutralized by the cancer cells. However, there are means of tapping into one's immune system to promote the recognition and destruction of cancer cells.

Sipuleucel-T (Provenge) is not on the list of "high-value Scrabble words," but is an important addition to the prostate cancer weaponry, approved by the FDA in 2010 for patients with progressive metastatic CRPC who are asymptomatic or minimally symptomatic. Provenge is a vaccine that fights prostate cancer by programming one's immune system to seek out and destroy prostate cancer cells. Although it can prolong life, it only rarely decreases PSA or reduces metastases.

Immune cells are filtered out from one's blood and exposed in the lab to cancer antigens and other chemicals that turn the immune cells into a vaccine. This vaccine is injected back into the body, where it causes an immune response to the cancer cells. Side effects are flu-like symptoms (fever, chills, muscle aches) that generally are self-limited.

Pembrolizumab (Keytruda) is a type of immunotherapy known as an immune checkpoint inhibitor. It was approved by the FDA in 2017 for use in patients whose prostate cancer demonstrates specific genetic mutations. It works by blocking immune-suppressive signals and activating tumor-killing cells. It is typically used only as a last resort after other treatments have been deemed ineffective. It is given intravenously once every three weeks. Although not all men have a favorable response to this drug, it can be highly effective in those who do respond, with marked reduction in PSA, tumor size, symptoms and progression.

Cytotoxic therapy ("cyto" = cells, "toxic" = poisonous)

Medical oncology is the specialty devoted to the use of cancer-killing medications, a.k.a. chemotherapy, to stop malignant cells from dividing, growing and spreading. Since chemotherapy is most effective for rapidly dividing cells and because many prostate cancers grow relatively slowly, chemotherapy is not usually a primary form of treatment as are surgery or radiation. All rapidly dividing cells are affected by chemotherapy—hair, skin, gastro-intestinal tract, testes, bone marrow. Although side effects can out-weigh benefits in the treatment of early prostate cancer, chemotherapy can be beneficial to treat pain and extend life in advanced prostate cancer.

When prostate cancer grows resistant to ADT, chemotherapy becomes a consideration. Chemotherapy is a systemic (as opposed to local) treatment that can control progressive growth and destroy prostate cancer cells that have become resistant to ADT. Although chemotherapy is usually used as a salvage treatment for CRPC or for metastatic prostate cancer, two recent clinical trials have demonstrated an improvement in overall survival using ADT plus chemotherapy (taxotere) in castrate-sensitive prostate cancer, prior to the development of resistance to hormonal therapy.

Taxotere (Docetaxel) was FDA approved in 2004 and when combined with prednisone has been the standard first-line chemotherapy for metastatic CRPC for many years. It can sometimes have a role in men with high volume prostate cancer that has not been managed with ADT. It alleviates pain, in-creases quality of life and increases survival. Side effects may include sup-pressed production of blood cells and platelets, fatigue, edema (swelling), neurological toxicity and changes in liver function. Historically, the stan-dard treatment prior to the Docetaxel era was mitoxantrone (Novantrone) combined with prednisone.

Cabazitaxel (Jevtana) is the newest addition to the chemotherapy weapon-ry. FDA approved in 2010, it is useful in prostate cancers resistant to other agents. Its primary toxicity is bone marrow suppression and for this reason it is almost always used in conjunction with a medication to boost infection-fighting white blood cells.

CRPC Management Challenges

Because of the recent availability of many new forms of treatment for CRPC, questions and controversies have arisen regarding benefits, risks and effects on quality of life, costs, use of single versus combined agents, optimal tim-ing (when to use) and sequencing (in what order to use) and how to best measure clinical benefits. For example, in patients with metastatic CRPC, treatment options include Zytiga, Xtandi, Erleada, Docetaxel, and Xofigo, all of which have different mechanisms of action and have been shown to pro-vide significant survival advantages. Management of CRPC continues to evolve and collaboration among urologist, radiation oncologist and medical oncologist will best determine optimal management.

Chapter 21: What is Genetic Testing for Prostate Cancer?

The last few years have witnessed a dramatic increase in our understanding of germline mutations as an important predisposing cause of aggressive prostate cancer. "Germline" mutations are those inherited DNA mutations that have existed since birth as opposed to "somatic" mutations that are mutations that have occurred after birth and are not passed on to children. About 10% of prostate cancers are thought to be on the basis of inherited germline mutations, the other 90% due to non-inherited, acquired mutations.

Germline mutations play a key role in many breast and ovarian cancers and it is now recognized that some of the same inherited germline mutations that increase the risk of these cancers in females—BRCA (BReast CAncer) mutations—can do the same in terms of risk for prostate cancer in men. BRCA1 mutations double the risk of metastatic castrate resistant prostate cancer (CRPC) and BRCA2 mutations increase the risk of metastatic CRPC by a factor of 4-6, with earlier onset, higher grade at diagnosis and shorter survival. More than 20% of men with metastatic CRPC are found to have germline mutations, the most common being BRCA2.

Germline mutation assessment (genetic testing) can help assess for prostate cancer risk whereas somatic mutation assessment (genomic testing), which closely examines the genes in a prostate cancer specimen, can help with decisions regarding treatment. Genomic testing can help predict how aggressively a prostate cancer might behave and how likely it is to advance and metastasize.

Genetic testing for prostate cancer is indicated in the following circumstances: early onset prostate cancer, aggressive prostate cancer, metastatic prostate cancer, in patients with multiple cancers that include prostate cancer (e.g. prostate cancer and male breast cancer) and in prostate cancer patients who have several family members with prostate, breast, ovarian, colorectal or pancreatic cancer.

Multigene panel testing uses either a blood or saliva sample to determine the presence of a panel of 14 genes commonly implicated in inherited prostate cancer. The most common mutations found are the BRCA2 mutation, which accounts for about 50% of hereditary prostate cancer mutations, and Lynch syndrome mutation. Lynch syndrome (hereditary non-polyposis colorectal cancer) is an inherited cancer syndrome causing mutations in DNA repair genes called MMR genes (MisMatch Repair). Because of this predisposition to mutation resulting from the impaired DNA repair, patients with Lynch syndrome have increased risk not only of colorectal cancers, but a host of other cancers including prostate cancer. Additional commonly found mutations are ATM (Ataxia Telangiectasia Mutation), HOXB13 (Homeobox B13) and CHEK2 (Checkpoint Kinase).

Chapter 22: What are Advanced Imaging Techniques?

Once the diagnosis of CRPC is made, it is important to use imaging studies to determine if metastases are present. Accurate staging provides guidance concerning the most appropriate form of treatment, which is targeted to the identified site of metastases. For many years, the best imaging methods for staging prostate cancer and detecting metastases were computerized tomography (CT) and nuclear bone scans. However, CT and nuclear bone scan have numerous limitations, although CT is useful in detecting the presence of advanced local disease (seminal vesicle invasion and invasion of surrounding local structures), enlarged lymph nodes and the presence of urinary tract obstruction. Bone scan has traditionally been the most widely used means of skeletal evaluation, often used for initial prostate cancer staging as well as for assessment for recurrence and metastatic disease. A limitation of the bone scan is false positives (bone scan shows abnormality in the absence of metastatic prostate cancer) that often require further imaging to sort out.

In recent years, more sophisticated and sensitive means of imaging prostate cancer have been developed and put into practice. The imaging studies available today include magnetic resonance imaging (MRI) and positron emission tomography (PET). MRI has shown value in defining local recurrence following surgery or radiation, particularly helpful in identifying extension of cancer beyond the prostate capsule and seminal vesicle invasion. PET scanning can detect early metastatic prostate cancer by identifying metabolic changes at the cellular level before they become evident on traditional imaging tests. Since the PET scan shows functional changes in the body, it is combined with CT imaging, which shows anatomical details, sites where the functional changes could be occurring. The combined PET/CT scan provides images that localize the abnormal metabolic activity.

PET scans use small amounts of chemicals that cancer cells require to grow and proliferate. These chemicals are "labeled" with radioactive materials. These labeled radiotracers are injected into the bloodstream where they are taken up to a greater extent in cancer cells than in surrounding normal cells. Any sites of recurrent cancer are identified as bright spots on imaging. These sites in men with a rising PSA following definitive treatment are commonly the prostate bed, lymph nodes and the bony skeleton.

Choline C11 PET/CT

Cancer cells have an enhanced demand for choline (part of the Vitamin B complex that becomes incorporated into cell membranes) to support their increased metabolism and proliferation. Choline C11 PET/CT uses choline labeled with a type of radioactivity called carbon-11 (C-11). The problem with choline C11 is its rapid rate of radioactive decay with its short half-life (20 minutes) restricting its use to centers that can produce the radiotracer on site or geographically close by.

Axumin (Fluciclovine F18 labeled synthetic amino acid analog) PET/CT

Cancer cells have an enhanced demand for amino acids (building blocks of proteins) to support their increased metabolism and proliferation. Axumin uses synthetic amino acids that are labeled with a type of radioactivity called fluorine-18. This test is particularly useful for detecting and localizing small recurrences of prostate cancer in men with rising PSA levels following treatment. The much more favorable half-life of F18 (2 hours) makes the Axumin PET/CT much more practical than the Choline C11 PET/CT.

Sodium fluoride (Na-F-18) PET/CT

Cancer cells that have metastasized to bones have an increased demand for certain growth factors and nutrients. Sodium fluoride PET/CT is a "bone-seeking" radiotracer that is taken up at sites of bone metastases more so than in surrounding normal bone cells, localizing the site and extent of bony metastases. It is a means of accurately detecting bone metastases in patients with advanced prostate cancer, an enhancement over traditional bone scans that can be used as a follow-up study when bone metastases are suspected but not definitive on bone scan.

Prostate specific membrane antigen (PSMA) PET/CT

"Prostate specific membrane antigen" (PSMA) is a protein found on the surface of prostate cells, normal or cancerous. It is over-expressed in prostate cancer tissue at all stages. PSMA expression is usually low in benign prostate enlargement, increased in prostate cancer and markedly increased with aggressive prostate cancer, CRPC, and metastatic prostate cancer. PSMA PET/CT uses small molecules that bind to prostate specific membrane antigen to enable improved staging and accurate detection of metastases in patients with advanced prostate cancer. It is one of the most promising of the different PET radiopharmaceuticals and is currently available in Europe and under clinical trial in the United States.

Chapter 23: What is Palliative Management?

Patients with advanced prostate cancer often value their quality of life as much as their quantity of life. "Palliative management," a.k.a. "supportive care," aims not to treat the advanced prostate cancer, but to provide comfort to the patient to improve their quality of life. This holistic approach addresses the patient as a whole and not just the disease. It includes management of pain from bone metastases, neurological issues that may result from bony compression of the spinal cord and/or nerves, and urinary tract obstruction. Efforts are directed at improving symptoms without curing the disease.

Localized bone pain

Patients with isolated bone metastases that are symptomatic typically have unrelenting, well-localized pain. The pain may be effectively treated with localized radiotherapy to the area of concern, often referred to as "spot radiation."

"Pathological" fractures—as distinguished from "traumatic" fractures—are broken bones due to bone weakness from normal cells having been replaced by cancer cells. If a pathological fracture from the prostate cancer involves a weight-bearing bone, orthopedic surgery (in addition to radiation) may be necessary to stabilize the bone. The most common pathological fracture site from prostate cancer is the hip.

As mentioned in the chapter on CRPC, **denosunab (Xgeva)** is a monoclonal antibody that effectively can delay skeletal related events. It has largely replaced Zometa because it is more easily administered (subcutaneous injection), does not have the same issues with kidney impairment, and has outperformed it in terms of effectiveness. Both medications rarely can cause jaw osteonecrosis (loss of bone integrity of the jawbone).

Diffuse bone pain

For patients who are symptomatic with extensive bony metastases, systemic radionuclide therapy using radiopharmaceuticals can be helpful. As discussed in the CRPC chapter, Xofigo is a radiopharmaceutical drug approved by the FDA in 2013 to treat bone-metastatic CRPC. It mimics calcium and forms complexes at areas of increased bone turnover. It contains the radioactive material radium 223, which works at the site of bone metastases, emitting radiation that has an anti-cancer effect. Because of a survival benefit in patients with symptomatic bone metastases as well as reduced bone marrow toxicity, Xofigo has largely replaced the previous generation radiopharmaceuticals Strontium-89 and Samarium-153.

Spinal cord compression

Spinal cord compression is a serious emergency for patients who have metastatic prostate cancer. The vertebral column can collapse when weakened by prostate cancer, compressing the spinal cord and/or nerves and leading to severe back pain, leg weakness, altered sensation, and bladder and bowel dysfunction. Even in the absence of vertebral collapse, the spinal cord and nerves can be affected by the presence of metastatic disease, causing pain and neurological symptoms.

Vertebral metastatic disease is an emergency that requires rapid evaluation with MRI imaging of the spine and treatment with high-dosage intravenous steroids and radiotherapy to the involved vertebra. Neurosurgical intervention may be necessary if there are progressive symptoms during radiation therapy or if there is a recurrence after radiation. If androgen deprivation therapy has not been previously used, it needs to be instituted immediately.

Urinary tract obstruction

Lower urinary tract obstruction can occur as the prostate cancer growth occludes the urethra (urinary channel from bladder neck to tip of penis). At times, this needs to be treated with surgery to create a channel through the obstruction to restore normal urinating.

Upper urinary tract obstruction can occur if the ureters (tubes that drain urine from the kidneys to the bladder) are compressed by local infiltration of the prostate cancer directly into the bladder base or by pathologically enlarged lymph nodes. This can be managed with "ureteral stenting" (placement of a small catheter within the ureter to alleviate the obstruction) or "percutaneous nephrostomy" (placement of a small catheter directly into the kidney from the flank to alleviate the obstruction).

Chapter 24: Bone Health and Prostate Cancer

Functions of bones

Bones comprise the foundation and scaffold that support the body. If the bony infrastructure is compromised, organs and tissues that depend on intact structural support can be negatively impacted. In addition to providing the body's framework, bones protect vital organs (e.g., the brain within the skull and the spinal cord within the vertebral column), allow for movement and mobility, and contain marrow that is responsible for production of the cellular elements of the blood. Additionally, bones are the reservoir for storage of minerals, particularly calcium and phosphate.

Bone mineralization

Bone consists of widely separated cells surrounded by a matrix of inorganic salts and collagen fiber. Bone mineralization—the process by which minerals are integrated into the matrix of bones—is a dynamic process since bones are not fixed in composition, but are continually being remodeled, restructured and refashioned. This occurs in accordance with the availability of component building materials in an adaptive response to biomechanical forces including gravity and muscular and skeletal stresses. "Osteoblasts" are the specialized cells that promote bone formation and "osteoclasts" are the cells that induce bone resorption.

Bone development

The bone formative process begins during childhood and continues through adolescence, when the body builds its greatest share of bone mass. Bone mass peaks in our early 20s. Like so many physical attributes, bone strength and integrity have a strong hereditary basis, although environmental factors are also important.

113

Environmental factors that contribute strongly to healthy bone development are diet, sun exposure, physical activity and maintaining a reasonable weight. Because calcium is a vital component of bone mass and vitamin D facilitates absorption of calcium, ample consumption of calcium and vitamin D are essential to develop and maintain healthy bones.

Calcium

A nutritionally-sound diet rich in calcium-containing foods includes dairy sources such as milk, yogurt and cheese. Non-dairy sources of calcium include vegetables such as Chinese cabbage, kale, broccoli and spinach. Seafood sources include salmon and sardines. Many food items are calcium-fortified, including breakfast cereals, tofu and fruit juices.

Vitamin D

Vitamin D, a fat-soluble vitamin that is stored in the liver and fatty tissues, is necessary to absorb and utilize dietary calcium. A brief amount of daily sunlight exposure is generally sufficient to ensure adequate levels of vitamin D, which the body manufactures in response to exposure to ultraviolet-B waves. Many people do not get sufficient sun exposure in winter months to make adequate levels of vitamin D since the sun is lower in the winter sky and exposure time is limited because of the cold weather and the need to bundle up in clothing. Vitamin D synthesis tends to diminish with age.

Exercise

Bones require physical activity to maintain their proper state of mineralization. Generally, the more active one is, the greater the bone mineral density (BMD) and the less risk for fracture. Most exercises promote bone health, but certain ones are better at achieving this than others. Just as our bodies require a variety of different and variable nutrients, so our bones demand a variety of different exercises, movements and stresses to maintain their health.

Fact: When our bodies are kept in a sedentary state—e.g., when one's arm is in a cast because of a fracture, or when one is immobilized by a severe injury and is at bed rest—there is rapid demineralization and thinning of the bones. Spinal cord injured patients who are paralyzed undergo a very rapid bone demineralization. Astronauts who spend time in zero gravity experience a remarkably fast demineralization and run the risk not only of thinning bones—as does anyone with rapid demineralization—but also of developing kidney stones that result from the calcium mobilized from the bones.

Bone mineralization is stimulated by varying stresses placed upon the bones, as opposed to repetitive, monotonous movements. BMD is greater in sprinters, ball sport athletes and gymnasts than in endurance sports athletes, including walkers, runners, swimmers and cyclists. Aerobic ball sport activities that provide variable stresses on bones that work against gravity and provide periods of rest include tennis, squash, football, soccer, basketball, hockey, field hockey, lacrosse, dancing and gymnastics. Additionally, weight training and any activity that uses resistance equipment can effectively promote bone mineralization. Physical training that involves straining, versatile movements, and high-peak forces more beneficially mineralize bone than training with many low-force repetitions.

Repetitive, unvarying stresses can demineralize bone and are an ineffective means of increasing bone strength. For this reason, runners and swimmers have the lowest BMD among athletes. Some studies have shown that endurance and non-weight-bearing sports participants may actually have bones that are weaker and at a greater risk of fracture than sedentary and inactive people. Endurance athletes may burn so many calories that there is insufficient energy remaining to fuel the process of bone health maintenance, with the possible consequence of stress fractures due to repeated strains on weight-bearing bones. To optimize bone health when running, swimming and cycling, it is best to do interval training at variable speeds, intensities and durations and not maintain monotonous motion. Of equal importance is sufficient calorie intake to fuel the bone mineralization process.

Body weight

Those with low body weight or who have recently experienced weight loss tend to experience more bone demineralization than those who are heavy. One of the few advantages of being overweight is that it requires extra effort to carry around the added pounds, and it is this exertion against the force of gravity that helps to mineralize and fortify bones.

Aging bones

There is a gradual loss of bone mass that occurs with aging, which correlates with the likelihood for "osteopenia," the medical term for bone loss. "Osteoporosis" is the medical term applied to severe bone loss, which incurs a greater risk of fractures.

Although osteopenia and osteoporosis occur in both genders, women are at much higher risk than men. The male and female sex hormones, testosterone and estrogen, respectively, promote bone health and mineralization. After menopause, with the sudden drop in estrogen there is typically an acceleration of bone loss. Men usually experience a gradual drop in testosterone levels with aging, with lower testosterone levels correlating with more bone loss. In general, men tend to experience bone loss at a slower rate than women since they weigh more and keep their bones better mineralized by supporting the extra weight; additionally, the testosterone decline with aging is much less than the accelerated decline in estrogen at menopause.

Prostate cancer and bone health

Prostate cancer in and of itself as well as its treatment can affect bone health and integrity. Patients with advanced prostate cancer are often older, a population at risk for less dense and more fragile bones. Additionally, these patients are often treated with androgen deprivation therapy (ADT) that further accelerates bone demineralization. Furthermore, bone metastases, not uncommon in advanced prostate cancer patients, also interfere with bone integrity and can give rise to pain, pathological fractures and spinal cord compression. Aging, ADT and bony metastatic disease create a perfect storm for poor bone health and bone-related skeletal events. Some men with advanced prostate cancer need to take steroids in conjunction with the medication used to treat the cancer (e.g., men on abiraterone and taxotere), which increases their risk for bone demineralization.

Bone metastases from prostate cancer are a state of increased bone turnover that involves the action of osteoblasts that form woven bone and osteoclasts that erode bone. Metastases largely consist of woven bone, which is structurally frail and increases one's risk of fracture. More than 80% of men with metastatic CRPC have bone metastases detectible on imaging tests. Metastases more typically involve the "axial "skeleton—vertebra, skull, ribs and pelvis—as opposed to the "appendicular" skeleton, which includes the long bones. Metastases to the vertebra can give rise to compression fracture and spinal cord compression as well as nerve root compression. Bone metastases can be evaluated with nuclear bone scans, although bone scans are non-specific and can "light up" for other reasons including old trauma, fractures, inflammation, infections and arthritis. The newer sodium fluoride (Na-F-18) PET/CT has been shown to be far more accurate than standard nuclear bone scanning.

Testing bone integrity

Bone mineral density can be measured and monitored using dual energy X-ray absorptiometry (DEXA) scanning, which uses a small dose of radiation to produce images of the lower spine and hips to quantitate bone loss. It is useful to diagnose osteoporosis and assess risk for fracture. Results are reported as T-score, the number of standard deviations from the mean that the measured bone loss differs from that of the mean of a young, normal population.

Bone-directed therapy

Men with bony metastatic CRPC are at increased risk for skeletal related events, including pathological fracture and spinal cord or nerve compression.

Prolia 60 mg every six months is used to help maintain bone integrity and limit loss of bone mass in men on ADT. **Xgeva** 120 mg every four weeks is used for men with rising PSA despite ADT or in metastatic CRPC patients to prevent skeletal related events. It decreases the risk of fractures and bone pain and delays the time to bone metastases. Prolia and Xgeva are the same drug, which works by inhibiting osteoclast activity. On rare occasions, they can cause osteonecrosis of the jaw.

Xofigo is a radiopharmaceutical drug used to treat minimally symptomatic or symptomatic metastatic CRPC requiring opioid or analgesic medication in men who have no significant lymph node enlargement and no spread to visceral organs. It mimics calcium and forms complexes at areas of increased bone turnover. It is given intravenously every 4 weeks, for a total of 6 doses. It contains the radioactive material radium 223, which works at the site of bone metastases, emitting radiation that has an anti-cancer effect and prolonging the time to the first skeletal related event. Xofigo can be absorbed by other organs, particularly those that are metabolically active, including bone marrow and the digestive system, which can result in anemia, low white blood cell count, low platelet count, bone pain, nausea, vomiting, diarrhea and swelling of the extremities.

Palliative radiotherapy can be used to relieve pain from metastases in metastatic spinal cord compression and in those with impending pathological fractures. At times, surgical decompression needs to be used for spinal cord compression and surgical stabilization for bone metastases that have a high risk of fracture.

Maintaining bone health in prostate cancer patients

Safeguards need to be taken to avoid the increased risk of bone fracture and other skeletal related events in prostate cancer patients. Although genetics, aging and gender are factors beyond one's control, intake of bone-building nutrients (calcium and vitamin D) and exercise are modifiable factors that are in our hands. All men on ADT should at minimum use a calcium and vitamin D supplement at the following recommended daily dose: 1200 mg calcium and 800-1000 units vitamin D3. Urologists often recommend **Prosteon** for men on ADT, a non-prescription supplement consisting of vitamin D3, vitamin K1, calcium citrate, magnesium oxide, strontium citrate and sodium borate (available through Theralogix.com). Sunlight exposure in moderation and participation in weight-bearing exercises and ball sports are helpful to maintain bone health and integrity in men with prostate cancer.

Chapter 25: Prostate Cancer Preventive Measures and Risk Reduction

If you are reading this book, chances are that you have already been diagnosed with prostate cancer. The advice that follows is relevant for men on active surveillance as well as for male children of prostate cancer patients and any men who desire to minimize their risk. It is equally applicable to men who have had their prostate cancer treated and wish to maintain a healthy life and minimize their chances of recurrence.

It would be wonderful if prostate cancer could be prevented and would certainly make my job much easier. Unfortunately, we are not there yet, but we have become wiser and more enlightened about measures that can be pursued to maintain health in general and help minimize the chances of developing prostate cancer.

Genetics, aging and race are factors that contribute to prostate cancer that are beyond one's control. However, environmental and lifestyle factors also play a role and can be influenced by positive behaviors. Healthy lifestyle and dietary practices can slow the growth and progression of prostate cancer just as unhealthy lifestyle and dietary practices can accelerate the growth and progression of prostate cancer.

Consider the fact that when Asian men—who have very low rates of prostate cancer—emigrate to western countries, their risk of prostate cancer increases over time. Clearly, a calorie-rich, nutrient-poor, Western diet overloaded with processed foods is associated with a higher incidence of many potentially preventable problems including prostate and other cancers as well as cardiovascular disease.

Not uncommonly, pre-cancerous lesions on prostate biopsy—high-grade prostate intraepithelial neoplasia (HGPIN) and atypical small acinar proliferation (ASAP)—predate the onset of prostate cancer by many years. This, coupled with the increasing prevalence of prostate cancer with aging, suggests that the process of developing prostate cancer takes place over a prolonged period of time. It is estimated to take many years—often more than a decade—from the initial prostate cell mutation to the time when prostate cancer manifests itself with either a PSA elevation, PSA acceleration or an abnormal digital rectal examination. In theory, this provides the opportunity for preventive measures and intervention before the establishment of a cancer.

Six Measures to Reduce Risk of Prostate Cancer (and reduce progression risk for men on active surveillance, those with pre-malignant biopsies, and those treated with conventional means)

A healthy lifestyle, including a wholesome and nutritious diet, weight management, regular exercise and the avoidance of tobacco and excessive alcohol, can lessen one's risk of all chronic diseases, including heart disease, diabetes and a host of cancers including prostate cancer. Good nutrition and an active lifestyle can not only reduce prostate cancer risk, but also slow progression.

1. **Maintain a healthy weight.** Obesity has been correlated with an increased risk for prostate cancer occurrence, recurrence, progression and death. Research suggests a link between a high-fat diet and prostate cancer. In men with prostate cancer, the odds of metastasis and death are increased about 1.3-fold in men with a body mass index of 30-35 and about 1.5-fold in men with a BMI > 35. Furthermore, carrying the burden of extra weight increases the complication rate following treatments for prostate cancer.

2. **Eat real food and avoid refined, over-processed, nutritionally-empty foods and be moderate with the consumption of animal fats and dairy.** A healthy diet includes whole grains and plenty of vegetables and fruits. Vegetables and fruits are rich in phytochemicals (biologically active compounds found in plants), including anti-oxidants, vitamins, minerals and fiber. Anti-oxidants help protect cells from damage caused by unstable molecules called free radicals, which can incur cellular damage and potentially cause cancer. Fruits such as berries (strawberries, blackberries, blueberries and raspberries), red cabbage and eggplant contain abundant anthocyanins, anti-oxidant pigments that give red, blue and purple plants their vibrant coloring. Tomatoes, tomato products and

other red fruits and vegetables are rich in lycopenes, which are bright red carotenoid anti-oxidant pigments. Cruciferous vegetables (broccoli, cauliflower, Brussel sprouts, kale and cabbage) and dark green leafy vegetables are fiber-rich and contain lutein, a carotenoid anti-oxidant pigment. A healthy diet includes protein sources incorporating fish, lean poultry and plant-based proteins such as legumes, nuts and seeds. Include fish rich in anti-inflammatory omega-3 fatty acids, e.g., salmon, sardines and trout. Processed meats and charred meats should be avoided. Healthy fats (preferably of vegetable origin, e.g., olives, avocados, seeds and nuts) are preferred. An ideal diet that is both heart-healthy and prostate-healthy is the Mediterranean diet.

"Let food be your medicine."
—Socrates

"Eat food. Not too much. Mostly plants."
—Michael Pollen

3. **Avoid tobacco and excessive alcohol intake.** Tobacco use has been associated with more aggressive prostate cancers and a higher risk of prostate cancer progression, recurrence and death. Prostate cancer risk rises with heavy alcohol use, so moderation is recommended.

4. **Stay active and exercise on a regular basis.** Exercise has been shown to lessen one's risk of developing prostate cancer and to decrease the death rate in those who do develop it. If one does develop prostate cancer, he will be in better physical shape and have an easier recovery from any intervention necessary to treat the disease. Exercise positively influences energy metabolism, oxidative stress and the immune system. Aerobic exercise should be done at least every other day with resistance exercise two to three times weekly. Pelvic floor muscle exercises benefit prostate health by increasing pelvic blood flow and lessening the tone of the sympathetic nervous system (the part of the nervous system stimulated by stress), which can aggravate lower urinary tract symptoms. Additionally, pelvic floor muscle exercises strengthen the muscles surrounding the prostate so that if one develops prostate cancer and requires treatment,

he will experience an expedited recovery of urinary control and sexual function.

5. **Be proactive and see your doctor annually for a DRE (digital rectal exam) and a PSA (prostate specific antigen) blood test.** The PSA test does not replace the DRE—both need to be done!

6. **Finasteride and dutasteride, commonly used medications to treat benign prostate enlargement, reduce the risk of prostate cancer.** These medications block the conversion of testosterone to its activated form—dihydrotestosterone (DHT)—that is responsible for prostate growth and male-pattern baldness.

The Prostate Cancer Prevention Trial was a clinical experiment that tested whether finasteride could prevent prostate cancer. This trial was based on the facts that prostate cancer does not occur in the absence of testosterone and that men born without the enzyme that converts testosterone to DHT do not develop either benign or malignant prostate growth (nor hair loss, for that matter).

This study enrolled almost 20,000 men who were randomly assigned to finasteride or placebo. The study was terminated early because men in the finasteride arm of the study were found to have a 25% risk reduction for prostate cancer.

The original study also demonstrated a slight increase in aggressive prostate cancer in the finasteride arm. This negative finding resulted in a "black box" warning from the FDA, as a result of which many men were frightened about the prospect of using the drug. However, long-term follow-up on the original clinical trial (presented at the 2018 American Urological Association meeting) concluded that finasteride clearly reduces the occurrence of prostate cancer and that the initial concerns regarding high grade prostate cancer were unfounded.

Prostates in those treated with finasteride were 25% smaller at the end of the study as opposed to the prostates in the placebo group. It is important to know that finasteride (and other medications in its class) lower PSA by 50%, so any man on these medications will need to have his PSA doubled to estimate what the PSA would be if not taking the medication.

Fact: When my thinning hair progressed to the point that I had a sunburn on my crown, I started using Propecia (a.k.a. finasteride). In a matter of a few years I had a full regrowth of hair. When the Prostate Cancer Prevention Trial report revealed a 25% risk reduction for prostate cancer with finasteride use, I was further motivated to continue using the drug, particularly since my father had been diagnosed with prostate cancer at age 65.

The bottom line is that finasteride (Proscar and Propecia) and dutasteride (Avodart) help prevent prostate cancer, shrink the prostate, improve lower urinary tract symptoms that are due to prostate enlargement, help avoid prostate surgery, and grow hair on one's scalp... a fountain of youth dispensed in a pill form! Furthermore, by shrinking benign prostate growth, these medications also increase the ability of the DRE to detect a prostate abnormality.

Chapter 26: Future Directions

Major research efforts and advances are being made in prostate cancer screening, detection, risk assessment, treatment and follow-up. Multiparametric MRI continues to evolve and the recent incorporation of more powerful magnets has resulted in more sophisticated device capabilities. Gene-based biomarkers and PET/CT imaging are in their infancy and show great promise in improving prostate cancer risk assessment and staging, respectively. Hundreds of ongoing clinical trials are exploring novel therapeutic strategies and investigational agents.

Focal therapies (HIFU, cryoablation, and focal laser ablation)—treatments directed at only the cancerous parts of the prostate gland—show potential but remain controversial because of the multifocal nature of prostate cancer and the lack of long-term outcome data. In select patients, focal therapy can offer an intermediate option between active surveillance at one extreme and active treatment (surgery or radiation) on the other.

The FDA has approved a host of new agents for advanced prostate cancer that potentially can increase life expectancy and prolong survival. The availability of so many options has made clinical decision-making more challenging, raising questions as to the most advantageous timing and sequencing of the different agents and the best combinations of agents to optimize treatment. These questions will be answered over the course of the next few years.

As opposed to chemotherapy that is cytotoxic and does not distinguish between normal and malignant cells, targeted medical therapies designed to treat only the prostate cancer cells are being explored. Ongoing trials include medications that inhibit the activity of growth factor receptors, those that interfere with the blood supply to prostate cancer cells, and those that stimulate the immune system to fight cancer cells. The emerging field of immunotherapy is an exciting new direction for prostate cancer, with great potential for checkpoint inhibitors/immune modulators (all have in common names that end in "-umab"), adoptive cell therapy and prostate cancer vaccines such as PROSTVAC, which activates the immune system to target PSA.

Advances in the branch of genomics concerned with the structure and activity of genetic material at the molecular level will play a pivotal role in the future. Genomic science has enabled the ability to determine the molecular "blueprint" of any given prostate cancer, the key to assessing its biological potential. By determining a cancer's unique genetic profile, it offers the potential for "precision medicine," individualized and customized treatment strategies with agents targeted against the specific mutations, a treatment based upon cancer biology and no longer only cancer histology.

12% of men with metastatic prostate cancer have germline mutations in genes that repair damaged DNA, accelerating the accumulation of mutations that ultimately cause the prostate cancer. Research is investigating drugs targeted to prostate cancers with mutations in these genes that repair damaged DNA, such as PARP (poly-ADP-ribose polymerase) inhibitors. Drugs that interfere with PARP-related DNA repair can create so many errors in prostate cancer cells that the prostate cancer cells die, an example of a medicine that uses the vulnerability of a cancer cell to destroy it. Recently, 63 new inherited DNA variants associated with increased prostate cancer risk have been identified, increasing the number of genetic risk regions to more than 170. Many of these newly discovered genetic variants are located in the sector of genes involved with communication among cells of the immune system, confirming the vital role of properly functioning immune pathways in decreasing prostate cancer risk.

> *"The signature of the tumor will allow us to fully assess the genetic nature of the enemy, how aggressive it is, what its metastatic intentions are, what it is sensitive to, and how best to attack it. At the same time, we will be armed with a whole battery of potent oral agents capable of targeting specific signaling pathways in the tumor."*
>
> *—Dr. Arie Belldegrun, Surgical Director of Genitourinary Oncology, UCLA School of Medicine*

Section II: Urinary Function

Chapter 27: Urinary Function After Prostate Cancer Treatment

In most circumstances, information about prostate cancer prognosis and treatment is adequately conveyed to the newly diagnosed patient. However, counseling and education about quality of life issues that may result from prostate cancer treatments are at times given short shrift or neglected. Insufficient attention is paid to these urinary and sexual side effects, perhaps understandable as being lower in the hierarchy of oncology priorities since prostate cancer is potentially a life-and-death issue. Urinary problems—particularly bladder control issues—can potentially be devastating, affecting psychological, emotional and sexual well-being and may be responsible for depression, loss of self-esteem and avoidance of activities that contribute to a healthy, productive and active lifestyle.

The intent of this chapter is to provide knowledge and realistic expectations concerning urinary function following the various treatments for prostate cancer. Although urinary issues are common consequences, they are manageable, and in most cases can be resolved, if not substantially improved.

Lower Urinary Tract Anatomy and Function

The bladder is a balloon-like muscular organ that stores and empties urine. The urethra is the tubular channel that conveys urine from the bladder out of the body. The innermost part of the urethra is surrounded by the prostate gland.

The urinary sphincters are the specialized valve-like muscles that surround the urethra and provide urinary control. The "main" sphincter is the internal sphincter, a.k.a. bladder neck sphincter, composed of smooth muscle and located at the neck of the bladder (where the urinary bladder and urethra meet). It is an involuntary muscle designed for sustained control and its location at the bladder neck gives it a mechanical advantage. The "assistant" sphincter is the external sphincter, a.k.a., striated sphincter, comprised of skeletal muscle and contributed to by the pelvic floor muscles and located below the prostate. It is a voluntary muscle that is situated downstream from the internal sphincter and is designed for emergency control. I liken the internal sphincter and the external sphincter to a car's brakes and emergency brakes, respectively.

The "guarding" reflex is a gradual increase in the contraction level of the external sphincter in direct relationship to the extent of filling of the bladder, a means of helping to maintain urinary control as bladder urine volume increases. The "cough" reflex is a contraction of the external sphincter that occurs with coughing, a means of helping to maintain urinary control when there is a sudden increase in intra-abdominal pressure.

The prostate envelops the urethra and is located between the bladder neck and external sphincter. The sphincters have an intimate anatomic relationship with the prostate gland, hence the potential for urinary control issues following prostatectomy.

The bladder is able to store urine by virtue of the fact that during bladder filling the bladder muscle remains relaxed at the same time that the sphincter muscles are contracted (squeezed). When the desire to urinate arises as the bladder fills to capacity (about 12 ounces), the coordinated contraction of the bladder muscle and relaxation of the sphincter muscles effectively empties the bladder.

Urinary Problems After Radical Prostatectomy

On a positive note, radical prostatectomy can alleviate obstructive and irritative lower urinary tract symptoms in men who have symptomatic benign prostate enlargement in addition to prostate cancer. Furthermore, men who undergo prostatectomy will never develop symptomatic benign prostate enlargement that many aging men will encounter and that often necessitates medication or surgery to improve their symptoms.

When the prostate is surgically removed, a gap is created between the bladder and the urethra. This gap is bridged by carefully sewing the bladder neck to the urethral stump, with a catheter left in the bladder for a week or so to facilitate the healing process. Most men who undergo surgical removal of the prostate will experience short term urinary incontinence immediately following catheter removal, since the surgery impacts the muscles and nerves responsible for urinary control. This incontinence will persist for the long term in only a small subset of men.

In most cases, the reconstructed connection between the bladder and urethra heals nicely, resulting in the preservation of bladder storage and emptying functions. However, at times the reconstructed connection can heal with scarring, which can cause urinary incontinence because of impaired sphincter function with the bladder neck scarred in a fixed and open position. When the internal sphincter is scarred in such a fixed and open position, it no longer has the elasticity and suppleness to provide the appropriate opening and closing necessary for urinary control. Urinary control then becomes dependent upon the external urinary sphincter. This auxiliary system is not designed for sustained contraction and although there is virtually constant tone to this muscle, only a relatively brief intense contraction can be achieved, insufficient to completely compensate for the dysfunction of the internal sphincter.

At other times, the reconstructed connection between the bladder and urethra heals in such a way that the scarring results in the bladder neck being in a fixed and narrowed position. The narrowing can give rise to obstructive lower urinary tract symptoms, including difficulty urinating with a hesitant, intermittent, weak stream, prolonged voiding time, the sensation of incomplete emptying and at times, the inability to urinate (urinary retention). This narrowing is referred to as a "stricture" or "contracture." When this problem is surgically addressed with a procedure to enlarge the narrowing by stretching or cutting into the scar tissue, the obstruction is relieved but urinary incontinence may result.

The main type of urinary incontinence that occurs after prostatectomy is stress urinary incontinence, urinary leakage associated with sudden increases in abdominal pressure as may happen with exercising, sneezing, coughing, bending, etc. The incontinence can be highly variable in degree, ranging from minor urinary volume leakage to major volume leakage that can occur with little provocation. Fortunately, for most men the situation improves, if not resolves completely over the course of the ensuing weeks, although at times it can take 6-12 months for full recovery.

Risk factors for urinary incontinence following prostatectomy are age (younger patients less incontinence), general health and body mass index (healthier and lower BMI less incontinence), extent of bladder control before the surgery (better pre-surgery control less incontinence), prior prostate surgery (more incontinence), skill of the surgeon and ability to do a nerve-sparing procedure (more skilled and nerve-sparing less incontinence), membranous urethral length (longer length less incontinence), stage (advanced stage more incontinence), adjuvant or salvage radiation therapy following prostatectomy (more incontinence), salvage prostatectomy following radiation therapy that has failed to arrest the prostate cancer (substantially more incontinence), and post-operative stricture requiring a procedure to fix it (more incontinence).

Of the men who never fully recover 100% of their urinary control, the resultant leakage is usually minimal and tolerable and tends to happen only when the bladder is full and during exercise or gravity-defying activities, such as bending over and standing upright. A small subset of men (less than 5%) may experience persistent, significant incontinence, a major quality of life issue that will need to be addressed.

Although stress urinary incontinence is the main type of incontinence that occurs after prostatectomy and other forms of prostate cancer treatment, other types of incontinence may occur as well. Urgency incontinence is leakage that occurs in transit to the bathroom associated with a strong sense of urgency, often on the basis of involuntary bladder muscle contractions. Overflow incontinence is a situation where the bladder leaks because it is overdistended with urine, as can occur with a stricture of the bladder neck. At times, urinary leakage can occur during sexual activities: foreplay, sexual intercourse and/or at the moment of sexual climax. Note that although medications can be highly beneficial for urgency incontinence, there is no effective pill to manage stress urinary incontinence.

Urinary Problems After Radiation Therapy

Urinary incontinence is less prevalent after radiation as compared to surgery. Surgical procedures done to address lower urinary tract obstructive symptoms following radiation therapy increase one's risk for urinary incontinence.

Urinary issues following radiation therapy can be subdivided into early-phase and late-phase. Acute (early-phase) urinary problems occur during and shortly after the radiation because of the prostate swelling and inflammation resulting from the ionizing radiation. The symptoms are similar to those of any inflammatory process of the bladder and are often temporary and will improve substantially, if not disappear completely, in time. Any preexisting lower urinary tract symptoms can be exacerbated from radiation, resulting in bladder irritation, urinary urgency, frequency, pain while urinating, difficulty urinating with straining and an intermittent urinary stream and perhaps urinary incontinence. Typically, within a few months following completion of the radiation therapy, resolution of the symptoms will occur.

Chronic (late-phase) urinary issues may sometimes occur years after completing radiation and are thought to be on the basis of radiation-induced alterations in bladder blood flow and scarring. This is known as radiation cystitis and can cause symptoms including blood in the urine, burning or painful urination, urinary frequency and difficulty urinating. Urinary bleeding due to radiation cystitis is oftentimes provoked by straining, particularly with bowel movements, as well as participation in vigorous activities. Cystoscopy (a visual inspection of the bladder with a narrow fiberoptic instrument) usually reveals a classic pattern of prominent, exuberant, vibrantly colored, tangled blood vessels. If the urinary bleeding does not respond to hydration and temporary restriction of activities, at times cauterization of the bleeding vessels will be necessary and is usually successful. If cauterization fails to stop the bleeding, other options can be used, including medications that can be placed into the bladder as well as hyperbaric oxygen therapy, in which 100% oxygen is administered in a total body chamber where atmospheric pressure is increased to enhance healing.

Urinary Problems After Focal Ablative Therapies (HIFU and Cryotherapy)

Ablative therapies result in the destruction of prostate tissue via heat or freezing, both of which can cause lower urinary tract symptoms because of tissue swelling and sloughing. Voiding difficulties following focal ablative therapies may occur because of passage of sloughed tissues or scar tissue causing urethral narrowing. Urinary incontinence can be a long-term complication. At times, dystrophic calcification may occur, a condition that results from chronic inflammation, tissue damage and tissue death. In this situation, the inner lining of the prostate becomes calcified and sometimes mechanically blocked from the presence of stones that form on chronically inflamed tissues.

Chapter 28: Pelvic Floor Training to Manage Urinary Issues After Prostate Cancer Treatment

Stress urinary incontinence—a spurt-like urinary leakage that occurs at times of increased abdominal pressure, as may occur with sports, coughing, sneezing, bending and other high impact activities—is a common occurrence immediately following prostatectomy. Since the resumption of urinary control is a gradual and incremental process, simple and conservative strategies should be tried before considering complex and invasive methods, a stepwise approach that generally provides excellent results. Pelvic floor muscle training is one of the principal conservative managements of urinary incontinence. Pursuing a pelvic exercise program starting before and continuing after prostate cancer surgery facilitates the resumption of urinary control. Pelvic floor contractions on-demand—briskly engaging the pelvic floor muscles immediately prior to any activity that triggers stress incontinence—can be highly effective.

Pelvic Floor Muscles (PFM)

The PFM are skeletal muscles comprised of both fast twitch and slow twitch muscle fibers. Fast twitch fibers predominate in high contractile muscles that fatigue rapidly and are used for fast-paced muscle action, e.g., sprinting. Slow twitch fibers predominate in endurance muscles, e.g., marathon running. The pelvic floor muscles have a baseline tone because of the presence of slow twitch fibers. The presence of fast twitch fibers allows their capacity for voluntary contraction. The PFM fibers are 70% slow twitch, fatigue-resistant, endurance muscles to maintain constant muscle tone (e.g., sphincter function and pelvic support) and 30% fast twitch, capable of rapid and powerful contractions (e.g., sexual climax, interrupting the urinary stream and tightening the anus). Aging causes a decline in the function of the fast twitch fibers but tends to spare the slow twitch fibers.

The deep pelvic floor muscles—a.k.a. levator ani muscle, comprised of the pubococcygeus, iliococcygeus and puborectalis muscles—form the bottom of the "core" group of muscles and comprise the floor of the pelvis. These muscles help support the pelvic organs, reinforce the external sphincter and, in conjunction with the sphincters, play an important role in maintaining urinary control.

When the internal sphincter is damaged, the bladder neck is often rendered in a scarred, fixed open position, similar to a brittle "washer" in a faucet that no longer has the elasticity and suppleness to provide closure. Under this circumstance, continence becomes largely dependent upon the external sphincter. Remember that the external sphincter is not designed for sustained contraction, as is the internal sphincter. Even though the external sphincter has a steady state level of tone to it, it can only be intensively contracted for a brief period of time on demand. A well-functioning external sphincter, in the face of a poorly functional internal sphincter—although helpful in combatting stress incontinence—does not provide sufficient "endurance" of closure to keep one completely dry. For this reason, men with stress urinary incontinence often report that the incontinence is better in the morning but becomes worse in the later afternoon hours, on the basis of external sphincter "fatigue."

Pelvic Floor Muscle Training

Since the external sphincter is a voluntary skeletal muscle that is contributed to by the levator ani, PFM training has the potential to increase its tone, strength, power and endurance. When this muscle complex is trained, the guarding and cough reflexes will become more robust to better maintain continence. PFM conditioning will hone the ability to produce a voluntary, sustained and powerful contraction to offset stress urinary incontinence.

Numerous clinical studies have shown the benefit of PFM training to facilitate an early return of urinary continence following radical prostatectomy. In addition to hastening recovery of urinary control, pelvic training has also been shown to improve the degree of incontinence and the severity of other lower urinary tract symptoms.

One needs to be attentive to the specific triggers that provoke the incontinence. By intensively contracting the pelvic floor muscles immediately prior to trigger exposure, the incontinence can be prevented, if not made less severe. For example, if the transition from sitting to standing is what brings about the leakage, a brisk and sustained pelvic muscle contraction during the process of standing up should help control the problem. This maneuver—engaging the pelvic floor muscles immediately prior to an activity that might provoke the problem—can be a highly effective means of managing stress incontinence and when practiced diligently, can ultimately become an automatic behavior.

I highly recommend the following exercise program as the most expedient means of achieving pelvic floor muscle conditioning, (disclaimer: I am co-creator of the program): PelvicRx (www.PelvicRx.com). It is a well-designed and easy to use, follow-along, interactive 4-week pelvic training DVD that offers strengthening and endurance pelvic floor exercises. It provides education, guidance, training, and feedback to confirm the engagement of the proper muscles. It is structured so that repetitions, contraction intensity and contraction duration are gradually increased over the course of the program. This progression is the key to optimizing pelvic strength and endurance in order to address urinary as well as sexual issues following prostate cancer treatment.

Ten Ways Of Knowing That You Are Properly Contracting Your Pelvic Floor Muscles

1. The base of your penis retracts inwards towards the pubic bone as you contract your PFM.

2. The testes rise towards the groin as you contract your PFM.

3. When you place your index and middle fingers in the midline between the scrotum and anus you feel these muscles tighten as you contract your PFM.

4. You can pucker your anus as you contract your PFM. The anus tightens and pulls up and in, known as the "anal wink."

5. You get a similar feeling as you do when you are ejaculating when you contract your PFM.

6. When you touch your erect penis, you feel the erectile chambers surge with blood as you contract your PFM.

7. You can make your erect penis elevate (lift and point) as you contract your PFM.

8. You can stop your urinary stream completely when you contract your PFM.

9. You can push out the last few drops of urine that remain after completing urination when you contract your PFM.

10. After pursuing PFM training you notice better urinary control (and the bonus of improved erections and ejaculation).

It is important to know that PFM conditioning is beneficial to ALL men, not just those who have had treatment for prostate cancer. The PFM are vital to male genital and urinary health and serve an essential role in sexual, urinary and bowel health. A fit and trained pelvic floor can help improve/prevent erectile dysfunction, ejaculation issues, stress urinary incontinence, overactive bladder, urinary after-dribbling and bowel urgency and incontinence.

Biofeedback

Biofeedback is an adjunct to PFM training that can be helpful in men who have difficulty in gaining an understanding of their PFM. Special sensors are used to relay auditory and visual feedback information about the quality and magnitude of one's PFM contractions. The intent of biofeedback is to enhance awareness of the PFM, ensure contraction of the proper muscles, and to optimize control over PFM function. Biofeedback is offered in the office setting by many urologists and pelvic floor physical therapists.

Pelvic Floor Physical Therapy

Physical therapy is commonly used to help rehabilitate injured muscles and joints prior to surgery, following surgery and as an alternative to surgery. Pelvic floor physical therapy is a sub-specialty of physical therapy that can be of great benefit to men with urinary control and other pelvic issues. It is a niche and growing specialty that provides an essential service for men who require pelvic rehabilitation therapy. On a simplistic basis, I liken pelvic floor physical therapists to personal trainers for the PFM, but they are so much more and can serve a vital role in the rehabilitative process.

Pelvic floor physical therapy can help effectively manage urinary incontinence, urinary urgency/frequency, sexual dysfunction and other pelvic issues that may follow treatment for prostate cancer. Pelvic floor physical therapists have extensive training in assessing strength, endurance, sensation, coordination and tone of the PFM. At the initial evaluation, the physical therapist examines muscles, connective tissue, joint mobility, nerve function, hip and spinal alignment and posture. PFM retraining enhanced with biofeedback is a key component of pelvic physical therapy. Patients are taught to coordinate the use of their PFM with functional activities including exercise, sitting, standing, home and daily activities, sexual intercourse, etc.

Chapter 29: Behavioral Management of Urinary Issues After Prostate Cancer Treatment

Behavioral modifications are simple, conservative strategies that target life-style, fluid consumption and voiding habits with the goal of improving urinary symptoms. These measures, although not curative, can reduce symptoms and improve quality of life. Since urinary control is a process that gradually and incrementally improves after treatment for prostate cancer, conservative options are sensible means that should be utilized before considering more invasive options.

Healthy lifestyle

Healthy eating and weight management are important since the burden of excess pounds can worsen urinary incontinence. Physical activities help maintain general fitness and lower impact exercises—yoga, Pilates, cycling, swimming, etc.—can boost core muscle (of which the PFM form the floor) strength, tone and endurance. Tobacco cessation can help improve urinary control since the chemical constituents of tobacco negatively affect bladder and sphincter function by constricting blood vessels and impairing blood flow, decreasing tissue oxygenation, promoting inflammation and contributing to coughing.

Moderation of fluid, caffeine and alcohol

Urinary incontinence will often not occur until a "critical" bladder volume is reached. By sensibly moderating fluid intake (but avoiding dehydration), it will take a longer time to achieve this threshold volume. Caffeine (present in tea, coffee, cola, some energy drinks and chocolate) and alcohol increase urinary output and can act as urinary irritants, so it is best to limit one's intake of these. Many foods—particularly fruits and vegetables—have significant hidden water content, so some moderation applies here as well.

Bladder irritants

Irritants of the urinary bladder may exacerbate urinary symptoms. Consider eliminating or reducing one or more of the following irritants and then assessing whether symptoms improve:

- Tobacco

- Alcoholic beverages

- Caffeinated beverages: coffee, tea, colas and other sodas and certain sport and energy drinks

- Chocolate

- Carbonated beverages

- Tomatoes and tomato products

- Citrus and citrus products: lemons, limes, oranges, grapefruits, citrus drinks

- Spicy foods

- Sugar and artificial sweeteners

- Vinegar

- Acidic fruits: cantaloupe, cranberries, grapes, guava, peaches, pineapple, plums, strawberries

- Dairy products

Medication assessment

Diuretic medications (water pills) can contribute to urinary incontinence. If on a diuretic, it may be worthwhile to check with your medical doctor to see if it is feasible to switch to an alternative, non-diuretic medication. This will not always be possible, but if a change to a different class of medication is made, there can be substantial symptomatic improvement.

Timed voiding (defensive voiding)

Urinating on a regular basis ("by the clock") before a sense of urgency occurs will keep the bladder as empty as possible. By emptying the bladder before a critical volume is reached, the incontinence can be controlled. Such "preemptive" or "defensive" voiding is a useful technique since purposeful and "voluntary" urinary frequency is more desirable than "involuntary" incontinence.

Bowel health

Avoidance of constipation is an important means of helping control urinary incontinence and other lower urinary tract symptoms. Because of the proximity of the rectum and bladder, a rectum full of gas or solid waste can put pressure on the bladder, resulting in worsening of urinary symptoms.

Chapter 30: Surgical Management of Urinary Issues After Prostate Cancer Treatment

Surgery is a consideration for treating the rare patient (about 4% of patients following radical prostatectomy) who has persistent, significant incontinence after sufficient time has passed to optimize healing and following failure of conservative management. Before embarking on surgery, it is imperative for the patient to undergo a comprehensive evaluation to determine the most appropriate treatment option and to be thoroughly counseled. This typically involves a cystoscopy to visually inspect the urethra, sphincters and urinary bladder and urodynamics to provide important information concerning bladder function. The type of surgical management needs to be tailored to the extent of the urinary incontinence as well as other factors, including the ability of the bladder to contract properly. The degree of incontinence is best quantified by pad usage, particularly by determining the weight of the pads used in 24 hours.

SURGICAL MANAGEMENT OF URINARY INCONTINENCE

Urethral Bulking Agents

Bulking agents are materials that are injected into the tissues around the urethra to "plump up" the urethra to help provide closure and improve urinary control. Injection of a bulking agent is a simple outpatient procedure that often needs to be repeated. Bulking agents currently available include carbon-coated beads suspended in a water gel (Durasphere) and silicone microparticles (Macroplastique).

The best results are achieved when injecting into healthy and supple tissue. However, many men with incontinence following prostatectomy have scarring of the bladder neck, making the tissues less receptive to bulking agents and accounting for the general less-than-satisfactory results. Many men who receive bulking agents will ultimately go on to either a male sling or artificial urinary sphincter. Since most patients do not achieve meaningful improvements in urinary control, urethral bulking agents are commonly used for short-term improvement in men who are poor surgical risks for more invasive treatments.

Male Sling

The male sling, although not as effective as the artificial urinary sphincter, is less invasive and incurs fewer potential risks and complications. Similar to a female urethral sling, a piece of supportive synthetic material (polypropylene) is strategically positioned underneath the deep, inner portion of the urethra via an incision in the area between the scrotum and anus. This provides control by creating either urethral compression or urethral relocation (support without compression) and is best suited for mild-moderate urinary incontinence as opposed to the artificial urinary sphincter that is used to manage severe urinary incontinence. Men who have received radiation therapy have poorer outcomes with sling implants than the non-radiated population and are better served by the artificial urinary sphincter. This is because radiation-induced scarring and fixation may limit the mobility of the urethra and the ability to relocate the urethra as well as interfere with tissue healing. Similarly, because of urethral scarring and fixation, men who have had a prior artificial urinary sphincter that has not been successful are not good candidates for a sling.

The array of slings available for the incontinent male include the trans-obturator sling (AdVance sling), the quadratic sling (VIRTUE) and an adjustable sling (Remeex). Success rates (0-1 pad daily) are moderate and complications include failure to improve the incontinence, inability to urinate, pain, infection, erosion and need for revision.

The trans-obturator sling relies on repositioning the urethra and thus requires an adequately mobile urethra that is not fixed and scarred. A fixed and scarred urethra is a situation that would be better served with a compressive means of management, including the quadratic sling or artificial

146

urinary sphincter. After tensioning the trans-obturator sling, it moves the urethra as much as an inch higher up in the pelvis and functions as a backboard during exertional activities, providing control as the increased abdominal pressure displaces the urethra into the backboard, pinching the urethra closed.

The quadratic sling is a four-armed mesh tape that relocates the urethra using a component that is placed via the groin and provides urethral compression using a component placed via the pubic area. Because this particular sling provides compression as well as relocation, it is best suited for men with a bladder that contracts normally as opposed to men with impaired bladder contractility (underactive bladder). An incontinent man who has impaired bladder contractility would be better served with a trans-obturator sling or artificial urinary sphincter. Because of the compression mechanism of action, the quadratic sling is better suited to men with more severe incontinence than would be able to be successfully addressed by the trans-obturator sling.

The Remeex adjustable sling consists of a short piece of mesh tape positioned under the urethra that is attached to a tensioning device placed in the pubic region. Sling tightening or loosening can be achieved by a minimally-invasive surgical means of accessing the tensioning mechanism.

Artificial Urinary Sphincter

The artificial urinary sphincter (AUS) is an effective, safe and reliable implantable medical prosthesis to restore urinary control in men with severe stress urinary incontinence that has not been suitably treated by other means. Although there is no way to totally replace one's natural sphincter system, the AUS is the only device that simulates normal sphincter function by opening and closing the urethra at the will of the patient. It provides consistent results in the treatment of incontinence following prostatectomy and is considered to be the "gold standard" in the management of this problem. Many patients report that the AUS is "life changing," converting bladder "cripples" back to normal function and restoring quality of life. About two-thirds of men will be completely continent after an AUS implant, and the other one-third will experience only minor incontinence, requiring one or two small pads per day. The overall patient satisfaction rate exceeds 90%. The AUS, first developed in 1972, has been used successfully for over 45 years and has been implanted in more than 150,000 men. Over the years, biomedical engineering refinements have further improved the AUS.

Severe involuntary leakage of urine following prostate surgery is a rare event, occurring in less than 5% of men following prostatectomy for prostate cancer. After prostatectomy, it most often results from scarring of the internal sphincter in a fixed open position. The AUS does not directly treat the damaged internal sphincter, but functions as a mechanical compression device of the urethra. The AUS is under the patient's command, providing simple and discreet control over bladder storage and emptying. Implanted entirely within the body, the device mimics the function of a healthy sphincter muscle by keeping the urethra closed until the patient desires to urinate.

The AUS is a hydraulic, saline fluid-filled device composed of solid silicone elastomer. It consists of three interconnected components: a cuff implanted around the urethra, a pressure-regulating balloon reservoir implanted behind the pubic bone adjacent to the bladder, and a control pump implanted in the scrotum. The cuff gently squeezes the urethra closed, preventing urine from passing. When one desires to urinate, he simply squeezes and releases the control pump that is situated in the scrotum, temporarily transferring saline fluid from the cuff to the pressure regulating balloon. The cuff opens, allowing urine to flow through the urethra and the bladder to be emptied. Within several minutes, the pressure regulating balloon automatically returns the saline fluid to the cuff to once again pinch the urethra closed.

In order to be an appropriate candidate for the AUS, the incontinence needs to be on the basis of a weakened or damaged sphincter and not due to bladder over-activity. Additionally, bladder capacity needs to be adequate and urinary flow rate sufficient to empty the bladder. The incontinence should be present for a minimum of 6 months before considering the AUS since spontaneous improvement occurs for some time after prostatectomy. One obviously needs to be sufficiently motivated to receive an implant, and its use demands manual dexterity in order to operate the control pump.

Implantation of the Artificial Urinary Sphincter (AUS)

Implantation of the AUS is an approximately one-hour outpatient surgical procedure done under anesthesia. The conventional operation is performed with one's legs in stirrups and requires one incision in the abdomen and another in the perineum (area between scrotum and anus). In 2003, Drs. Steve Wilson, John Delk, Gerard Henry and I devised an innovative technique for AUS implantation via a single scrotal incision. The advantages of the scrotal technique are a single incision (versus two incisions), the fact that it can be done supine, which is an easier position to work with (versus legs up in stirrups), faster operative time, ease of doing the procedure and decreased patient discomfort. In either case, the control pump is one-size-fits-all, but the cuff is precisely measured to one's anatomy and the pressure-regulating balloon reservoir is usually chosen to be 61-70 cm water pressure.

It is important to know that following implantation the AUS is not activated—and thus will not be functional—for about a 6-week period of time to allow for healing of tissues. Activation is a simple office process involving minimal discomfort.

It is advisable to order and wear a MedicAlert bracelet (www.medicalert.org) to inform health care personnel that you have an AUS implant in the event of a medical emergency. If you were rendered unconscious or unable to communicate, this bracelet will inform emergency medical staff that you have an AUS, because if there is ever a need for placement of a urethral catheter, it is imperative that the AUS be deactivated prior to catheter placement in order to avoid damaging the urethra.

FAQ

Who manufactures the AUS?

American Medical Systems Men's Health Division of Boston Scientific, Inc.

Will insurance cover the AUS?

Medicare has a coverage policy for incontinence control devices, which includes the AUS. Most commercial health insurers also cover the AUS when deemed medically necessary for the patient.

How effective is the AUS?

More than 90% of patients with the AUS have greatly improved continence, many of whom achieve complete urinary control with no need for pads and the remainder of whom have occasional, minor stress incontinence with vigorous activities, typically requiring one or two small pads per day. The commonly implanted pressure regulating balloon provides 61-70 cm of pressure around the urethra, which is sufficient closure for most of the activities of daily living.

Does the AUS need to be measured to my body?

The control pump is one-size-fits-all, but the cuff is sized to the circumference of your urethra to achieve a proper fit. The reservoir comes in a variety of pressures. The higher the pressure of the reservoir, the tighter the closure of the urethra. The tighter the closure of the urethra, the better the continence, but also the greater the chance of urethral damage from the higher pressures. A balance must be achieved in order to achieve the necessary pressure to achieve continence while minimizing potential damage to the urethra. In practical terms, this translates into a 61-70 cm pressure reservoir for most men.

Can I have an AUS if I underwent surgery followed by radiation therapy?

Yes, but radiation therapy increases the potential risk for complications because of tissue damage, scarring, decreased blood flow and less optimal wound healing.

Who should not have an AUS?

The AUS is not appropriate for a man with an obstructed lower urinary tract. It also should not be used for those with bladder-related incontinence (overactive bladder or a small-capacity, scarred bladder) as it is indicated only for those with sphincter-related incontinence. It cannot be effectively used in those with compromised dexterity or mental acuity.

What are the potential risks and complications of AUS implantation?

Infection   As with any surgery, an infection can develop after an AUS implant. Every step is taken to reduce the likelihood of an infection, including use of intravenous antibiotics, an antiseptic scrub of the surgical site followed by the application of a chlorhexidine and alcohol skin antiseptic immediately prior to the operation, double-gloving, meticulous surgical technique with the procedure done in the least amount of time as feasible, topical antibiotics to flush the surgical site, and minimizing operating room traffic. Antibiotic ointment is placed on the surgical incision prior to placing the surgical dressing. Patients are sent home with oral antibiotics.

Two of the three components of the AUS–the cuff and pump–are coated with an antibiotic combination called InhibiZone, which consists of rifampin and minocycline.

If an infection occurs and does not respond to antibiotics, it may be necessary to remove the AUS, an extremely rare occurrence.

Erosion   This is a breakdown of the urethral tissues that lie beneath the cuff. It is generally treated with cuff removal to allow for urethral healing prior to consideration for cuff replacement at a later date. Erosion can occur when a catheter is placed into the urinary bladder by health care personnel uninformed that the AUS device is in place. The delicate urethra, pinched closed by the inflated cuff surrounding it, is traumatized and damaged by catheter placement. This situation can be avoided by deactivating the AUS prior to catheterization. This is one of the reasons that a Medic-Alert card and bracelet are useful considerations. Erosion of the other AUS components can also occur on a rare basis. The control pump can potentially erode through the scrotal skin and the pressure-regulating balloon reservoir into the urinary bladder.

Mechanical Malfunction   The AUS device is effective and reliable, but like any mechanical device, it can ultimately malfunction. It is not possible to predict how long an AUS will function in an individual patient. As with any biomedical prosthesis, the device is subject to wear, component disconnection, component leakage, and other mechanical problems that may lead to the device not functioning as intended and that may ultimately require additional surgery to replace the device. The median durability of the device is about 7.5 years, although I have patients who still have a functional AUS twenty years following implantation.

Urethral Tissue Atrophy   This may result from the long-term pressure effect of the cuff on the urethra. Essentially, the urethra shrinks down from being squeezed by the cuff, resulting in gradual worsening of urinary control. When this happens, it generally requires repositioning of the cuff to a new urethral location or the use of a smaller cuff or, on rare occasions, placement of a second cuff (tandem cuff).

Pain   Discomfort in the groin, penis, scrotum and perineum is expected immediately after surgery and during the period when the device is first used. It is very rare to experience chronic pain from an AUS implantation.

Migration and Extrusion   Migration is movement or displacement of AUS components within the body space in which they were originally implanted. Extrusion occurs when a component moves to an abnormal location outside of the body. These are both extremely rare occurrences.

Chapter 31: Supportive Measures (Pads, Undergarments, External Collection and Penile Compression Devices)

Urinary incontinence can often be significantly improved or cured with pelvic floor muscle training, behavioral treatments and surgery. However, there are times when incontinence cannot be satisfactorily addressed by these means and certain circumstances for which surgery is not a feasible consideration. In some situations, only a simple and basic management is desired. The following is a brief review of absorbent pads, padded undergarments and external urinary collection and compressive devices.

Note: Many of the products discussed below can be purchased online at the Urology Health Store (www.UrologyHealthStore.com)

Pads and undergarments

There are many incontinence products available at drugstores, supermarkets, medical supply stores and online. These items have in common the ability to absorb urine and wick it away from the skin. The choice of product is usually based upon the extent of the urinary incontinence. The gamut of products includes absorbent padded sheaths that fit around the penis (drip collectors), pads placed within the underwear, cup-shaped guards, incontinence briefs and absorbent underwear, some of which are disposable and others of which are washable.

External collection devices

These are latex or silicone condom-like devices that are placed on the shaft of the penis and are secured to the penis with an adhesive. They drain via tubing into a urine collection bag.

Compression devices

These devices have in common a pinching mechanism that is applied to the urethra, similar to squeezing one's penis to prevent urinary leakage. The goal is to stop the incontinence while not compromising penile blood flow and maintaining a reasonably comfortable fit. Only minimal pressure on the urethra is required to stop urinary leakage. There are many such devices on the market. The devices that are discussed below work by applying compression pressure to the penis and with the exception of the Urostop device are worn just behind the head of the penis. They are removed for urinating and should not be worn while sleeping.

Cunningham clamp is a foam-padded metal clamp that comes in a variety of sizes. The pressure is regulated by spring wire loops that can be ratcheted into 5 different settings.

Baumraucker clamp is a foam-padded clamp similar to the Cunningham clamp, but has no metal parts and uses Velcro to secure the closure.

Dribblestop is a foam-padded, lightweight plastic device consisting of two clamps held together by adjustable links (of 3 varying lengths) to calibrate the urethral compression. The compression can be further fine-tuned by choosing one of two notches on the clamps.

Regain is a flexible plastic compression device that wraps around the penis and is available in 3 sizes. It consists of two arms connected by a hinge in the middle. A control pad is present on the inner surface of the lower arm and the upper arm is attached to a Velcro wrap-around strap. The penis is placed through the central opening and the device is hinged to envelop the penis. The elastic strap is wrapped around to hold the device in place and to apply urethral pressure.

Acticuf is a disposable pouch that contains an absorbable pocket. It has a mouth that opens to allow placement of the penis within the pouch. The pouch functions to collect and absorb urine and the mouth to compress the urethra. It can be loosened up by squeezing and releasing the compression mechanism a few times. It should be repositioned every 3-4 hours or so and not worn while sleeping and should be removed and discarded when saturated.

Urostop is used for preventing urinary leakage that occurs with sexual activity, whether during foreplay, intercourse or climax. It is an adjustable tension silicone loop that is placed at the base of the penis prior to sex and cinched down to occlude the urethra. The device should not be left on for more than 30 minutes.

Section III: Sexual Function

Chapter 32: Introduction to Male Sexual Function

Sex is a vital aspect of human existence—instinctual, hard-wired and a biological imperative. Nature has created the ultimate "bait and switch" in which reproduction (procreation) is linked with a pleasurable physical act (recreation), ensuring mating and, ultimately, perpetuation of the species.

Healthy male sexual function entails possessing a good libido (sex interest and drive), the ability to obtain and maintain a rigid erection, the capacity to ejaculate, experience a climax and to satisfy one's partner. Regardless of whether a man is sexually active or not, he usually relishes the capability of functioning sexually the way nature intended.

The impact of sexuality extends beyond the bedroom, contributing to masculine identity and behavior and inciting a "swagger" that permeates positively into many areas of a man's life. There is good reason why "cocksure" means "possessing a great deal of confidence." Although sex is by no means a necessity for a healthy life, the loss or impairment of sexual function can result in embarrassment, isolation, frustration and depression. An inoperative or poorly operative penis often results in the feeling of being "unmanned" and emasculated. This can be ego-deflating and negatively impact self-esteem and be detrimental to other aspects of a man's life, as well as give rise to many undesirable partner issues.

Long after the reproductive years are over and fatherhood is no longer a consideration, most men still wish to be able to achieve respectable enough erections to have sexual intercourse. However, the ravages of time, poor lifestyle habits, and medical issues and their treatment can wreak havoc on penile anatomy and function.

Prostate cancer and its treatment can adversely affect erections and ejaculation because of the intimate anatomical relationship between the prostate and the nerves involved in erections and since the prostate is a reproductive organ that contains the ejaculatory ducts. This problem is compounded by the fact that many men who are diagnosed with prostate cancer are older and have compromised erectile function predating the cancer diagnosis, and furthermore, have partners who often have sexual issues of their own.

"But the wheel of time turns, inexorably. True rigidity becomes a distant memory; the refractory period of sexual indifference after climax increases; the days of coming are going. Sexually speaking, men drop out by the wayside. By 65, half of all men are, to use a sporting metaphor, out of the game; as are virtually all ten years later, without resort to chemical kick-starting."

—Tom Hickman, God's Doodle: The Life and Times of the Penis

Chapter 33: Sexual Function After Prostate Cancer Treatment

In most circumstances, information regarding prognosis and treatment of prostate cancer is adequately communicated to the newly diagnosed patient. However, counseling and education about quality of life issues that may result from prostate cancer treatments are at times marginalized or neglected. Sexual dysfunction is one such sidelined issue, perhaps understandable as being lower in the hierarchy of oncology priorities since prostate cancer is potentially a life-and-death issue. Nonetheless, sexuality is vital to the well-being of many men and sexual dysfunction is the most common quality of life complaint in prostate cancer survivors. All management options for prostate cancer—active surveillance excluded—incur the potential risk of sexual issues.

Some physicians are uncomfortable addressing and discussing sexual dysfunction, whereas others do not consider themselves adequately trained to do so. Some patients feel ashamed or embarrassed to ask questions about sexuality after treatment or may regard sexual dysfunction as an inevitable and acceptable side effect in the face of a serious cancer.

Prostate cancer patients and their partners are entitled to be informed about potential adverse sexual side effects of treatment and provided with realistic expectations regarding their sexual functioning after treatment. The intent of this chapter is to provide knowledge about the sexual issues that may result following the various treatments for prostate cancer. The chapters that follow address how these sexual issues can be effectively managed.

In certain circumstances, prostate cancer itself can give rise to sexual dysfunction. Locally advanced prostate cancer can directly invade the all-important-to-erections neurovascular bundles that are situated in close proximity to the prostate. Advanced prostate cancer that has spread to the vertebral column can cause compression of the spinal cord and nerves that may give rise to a host of neurological problems, including sexual issues.

Most of the time, however, it is not the presence of prostate cancer that causes sexual dysfunction, but rather the side effects of the treatment. Patients who undergo surgery, radiation, androgen deprivation therapy and focal ablative therapies commonly experience impairments in sexual function and sexuality. High levels of sexual "distress" may be associated with the sexual dysfunction following treatment, marked by concern, anxiety, frustration, feelings of inadequacy and other negative emotions.

Because of the prostate's location—in a busy sector at the crossroads of the urinary and reproductive tracts, connected to the bladder on one end, the urethra on the other, touching upon the rectum, and nestled behind the pubic bone in a well-protected nook of the body—its surgical removal or treatment with radiation or focal therapies has the potential for causing undesirable side effects. Although urinary and sexual functions are discrete and separate, their interplay is complex and this distinction can be muddled by treatment modalities. The paired bundles of nerves and blood vessels (neurovascular bundles) that provide the nerve supply to the erection mechanism are delicate, intimately attached to the prostate gland, and can easily be traumatized by prostate cancer treatments as can muscles surrounding and supporting the prostate, resulting in altered sexual function and urinary control. Since the nerves are responsible for relaying the message to the penile arteries to expand and fill the erectile chambers of the penis with blood, if one is "unnerved" by surgery, radiation or other treatments, erectile consequences are likely to follow.

There are four basic components of male sexual function, all of which can be affected by prostate cancer treatments: Libido (sex drive); erections; ejaculation; and orgasm.

Although libido is complex and multifactorial, it is chemically driven by the hormone testosterone. Androgen deprivation therapy achieves castrate levels of testosterone, which drastically reduces one's interest in sex. Additionally, poor quality or absent erections as a side effect from prostate cancer treatments or due to other reasons can secondarily diminish libido, as one tends to lose interest in endeavors that cannot be successfully achieved. Other factors influencing libido are stress, fatigue, anxiety, depression and relationship issues, all of which can be affected by the diagnosis and treatment of prostate cancer.

Erectile rigidity and durability can be adversely affected by prostatectomy, radiation and other therapies. Lack of or diminished erections can perpetuate erectile dysfunction because of a "use it or lose it" phenomenon with the need for ongoing erections to maintain health and integrity of the penile tissues. (More about this later in a separate chapter.)

Ejaculation is the physical aspect of sexual climax in which semen is expelled by rhythmic contractions of the pelvic floor muscles. Erections and ejaculation are wired independently in the nervous system and thus it is possible to experience ejaculation even in the absence of an erection. Ejaculation after prostatectomy is "dry" because of the removal of the ejaculatory apparatus, including the prostate gland, seminal vesicles and the ejaculatory ducts. Even though no semen is ejaculated, the sensation of release is often preserved, although it may be different than before the surgery. At times, a consequence of prostatectomy can be leakage of urine with sexual stimulation and/or ejaculation of urine at the time of sexual climax. Radiation therapy commonly results in diminished to absent ejaculation volumes and can also cause an altered quality of ejaculation.

Orgasm is the psychological and emotional aspect of sexual climax that takes place in the brain. Although orgasm is possible even with the reproductive organs removed or irradiated, it may be of a different quality and intensity than prior to the treatment.

SEXUAL ISSUES AFTER PROSTATECTOMY

As a result of the high survival rates following treatment for prostate cancer, after concerns and fears about the cancer are gone or greatly diminished, side effects that affect quality of life achieve greater significance and become "front burner" issues. Although the initial grieving process concerned the diagnosis of prostate cancer, once the disease is addressed a new grief can surface for patient and partner—worry, anxiety, distress, frustration, despair and even depression—over the resulting impairment of sexual function.

Erectile dysfunction and dry ejaculation are the most common adverse sexual effects experienced after prostatectomy. Other sexual effects that may be encountered include the following: urinary leakage with foreplay and sexual stimulation; ejaculation of urine at the time of sexual climax; altered sensation of sexual climax; pain with sexual climax; penile shortening and deformity; and Peyronie's disease.

The potential psychological impact of sexual side effects following prostatectomy cannot be understated. Changes in urinary and sexual function can have a profound effect on psychosocial function, masculine identity and self-esteem, impacting one's partner as well as one's relationship with their partner.

Erectile dysfunction

Many men prior to prostate cancer treatment had experienced daily erections, and had done so for the entirety of their lives. However, immediately following prostatectomy, erections often halt abruptly. Understandably, in many men this generates major concerns about their sexuality. Another source of male anxiety that emerges is apprehension about their ability to satisfy their partner. Fortunately, despite the importance of sex for many couples, intimacy can be equally important to, if not more so, than sex. Furthermore, all forms of sex can be enjoyable and there are numerous ways one can sexually satisfy one's partner aside from penetrative penile-vaginal intercourse. Both partners are capable of achieving sexual gratification and climax without the involvement of an erect penis.

To compound the issue, both the prostate cancer patient and his partner are often in the age group where sexual dysfunction is common, with "andropause" (a controversial term referring to the gradual decline in testosterone levels experienced at midlife and beyond) and menopause, respectively, affecting their sexual health. The female partners of men treated for prostate cancer are often post-menopausal and experience parallel issues that affect sexuality—decreased libido, vaginal dryness and irritation, insufficient lubrication, vaginal narrowing and shortening, painful intercourse, urinary incontinence, pelvic organ prolapse, etc. The positive side to this is that the sexual issue is mutual and shared, but the negative side is that having both parties compromised negatively impacts the couple's ability to have sexual intercourse since it "takes two to tango." The recently introduced concept of "couple-pause" strives to address the sexual needs of the couple as a whole—a couple-oriented approach—rather than treating each partner in isolation.

The prostate does not directly contribute to the ability to obtain and maintain an erection, so its removal per se does not inevitably mean erectile dysfunction. However, the prostate is surrounded by nerves and blood vessels that are vital for normal erectile function, and it is the injury to these that fosters the erectile dysfunction.

Unquestionably, there are men who undergo prostatectomies performed by skilled robotic urologists who experience no complications whatsoever, achieving "trifecta" status: undetectable PSA, full urinary control and intact erectile function (although the recovery process can be lengthy and require the assistance of penile rehabilitation techniques). That stated, regardless of whether the prostatectomy spared the nerves or not, erectile dysfunction remains the leading post-operative complication, caused by damage to the delicate neurovascular bundles and tying off of the accessory arterial supply to the penis. The vast majority of men after prostatectomy will experience erectile dysfunction, many of whom will recover function. Clearly, the best post-operative erectile function will occur in younger men, those with excellent erectile function preceding the surgery, and in those who undergo a bilateral nerve sparing procedure performed by a skilled and experienced surgeon.

The "acute" erectile dysfunction following prostatectomy that is a consequence of the temporary loss of nerve conduction—a.k.a. "neuropraxia" in medical speak—can ultimately result in "chronic" erectile dysfunction. The lack of nerve transmission results in a constantly flaccid penis with poor oxygen flow to the erectile tissues. In a vicious cycle, erectile smooth muscle cells are replaced with collagen (scar tissue) resulting in further impairment of function with loss of the mechanism that ensures blood trapping in the erectile chambers. This venous leak from the erectile chambers impairs both erectile rigidity and durability. The bottom line is that future erections demand current erections, since erections are needed to maintain the health, tissue integrity and function of the erectile tissues. (More about this in the chapter "Use It or Lose It.")

Dry ejaculation

Although there is no release of semen following removal of the prostate gland, seminal vesicles and ejaculatory ducts, one is still capable of feeling the sensation, muscle contractions and pleasure experienced prior to surgery. The absence of ejaculation can be disturbing to some men, younger men in particular.

All patients following prostatectomy lose the ability to father children. If one wishes to retain fertility following prostatectomy, it is important to talk to his urologist about the possibility of banking sperm in advance of the surgical procedure. Sperm banking involves freezing semen in liquid nitrogen and storing it for future use with assisted reproduction techniques such as in vitro fertilization. Alternatively, since the testes continue to produce sperm for a number of years, testicular sperm aspiration (removing sperm cells using a tiny needle) with in vitro fertilization is another possibility.

Urinary leakage with sexual stimulation

Urinary leakage can sometimes occur with sexual foreplay, potentially an embarrassing issue for both patient and partner. This most commonly occurs during the first year after surgery and thereafter tends to improve. Potential solutions include pelvic floor muscle training, emptying one's bladder completely before engaging in sexual activity, and using either a condom that will collect any leaked urine or a penile constriction loop that compresses the urethra.

Ejaculation of urine

Although ejaculation is typically dry after prostatectomy, it is estimated that at least 20% of men may ejaculate some urine at the time of sexual climax. The actual number of men who experience this may be even greater because of a "no ask" and "no tell" phenomenon in which doctors are reluctant to ask about the problem and patients are reluctant to bring up the problem.

Even though the ejaculation consists of urine and not semen, the sensation at climax is often the same. Urine is generally sterile, so there is limited potential for spreading an infection to a partner. However, this "climacturia" as it is known in medical speak can be a nuisance and a source of embarrassment for both patient and partner and is a significant impediment that may lead to avoidance of sexual intimacy.

It typically is most prevalent during the first year after prostatectomy and thereafter tends to improve. Coping strategies are urinating immediately prior to engaging in sexual activity and using a condom or a constrictive penile loop, as are used for urinary leakage with foreplay and sexual stimulation. Pelvic floor muscle training has been shown to help this issue. If this situation does not respond well to conservative means, the male sling can be an effective means of management.

Altered climax

Sexual climax after prostatectomy may feel different than before the surgery. Some men feel a diminished sense of pleasure and intensity. In others, the dry ejaculation negatively impacts their perception of orgasm. In some men, sexual climax does not occur at all. A small percentage of men experience more intense orgasms than before the surgery. Overall, the most influential factors that are predictive of which men will have better preserved orgasmic function following prostatectomy are the following: extent of nerve preservation (better with nerve sparing), the extent of lymph node sampling (worse with more extensive sampling), age (younger better), and time elapsed since prostatectomy (more time better).

Painful climax

After prostatectomy, some men will experience discomfort or pain with sexual climax, which can be perceived in the penis, testes, perineum or rectum. In time, both the intensity and frequency of pain usually diminish, although a fraction of men may have persistent pain that persists beyond several years.

Penile changes

After prostatectomy, it is not uncommon to experience decreased penile length and/or girth. This shrinkage occurs during the first several months after the prostatectomy. The shortening is likely based on several factors. The gap in the urethra (because of the removed prostate) is bridged by sewing the bladder neck to the urethral stump, with a consequent loss of length from a telescoping phenomenon. Traumatized and impaired nerves and blood vessels vital for erections cause acute onset of erectile dysfunction. Thereafter, the lack of regular erections results in less oxygen delivery to penile smooth muscle and elastic fibers resulting in scarring, shortening and narrowing of the penile tissue, a phenomenon referred to as "disuse atrophy."

Resuming sexual activity as soon as possible after surgery will help "rehabilitate" the penis and prevent disuse atrophy. There are a variety of effective penile rehabilitation methods to help avoid disuse atrophy and to help get one "back in the saddle," to be discussed in detail in the chapters that follow.

Peyronie's disease

Fact: Peyronie's disease is named after the French surgeon, Francois Gigot de la Peyronie, who first described it in 1743.

Peyronie's disease, an acquired deformity of the penis, has been reported to occur in up to 15% or so of men after prostatectomy. It occurs due to scarring of the sheath of the erectile chambers, resulting in findings that may include the following: a hard lump, penile shortening, curvature with erections, penile narrowing, a visual indentation that can be described as an "hour-glass" deformity, pain with erections and decreased erectile rigidity. Penile pain, curvature and poor expansion of the erectile chambers contribute to difficulty in having a functional and anatomically correct rigid erection suitable for intercourse. Although the scarring is physical, it often has psychological ramifications, causing anxiety and depression.

During "acute" Peyronie's disease, erections are painful and there is an evolving scar, curvature and deformity. The "chronic" phase occurs up to 18 months or so after initial onset, at which time the pain and inflammation resolve, the curvature and deformity stabilize and erectile dysfunction is often noted. Treatment options include oral medications, topical agents, penile traction therapy, low-intensity shock wave therapy, injections of medications directly into the scar tissue and a variety of surgical managements, depending on circumstances.

SEXUAL ISSUES AFTER RADIATION THERAPY

Erectile dysfunction is the most common long-term side effect following radiation therapy (external beam radiation and brachytherapy), occurring in about 30-40% of men, regardless if the most recent iteration of image-guided radiation therapy was used. Radiation leads to changes in erectile tissues, including small blood vessel obliteration, tissue atrophy and scarring.

Whereas the decline in erectile function is immediate after prostatectomy with gradual improvement and a delayed recovery that can take 2 years or longer, erectile dysfunction after radiation therapy has the opposite trajectory—a slow and gradual decline over 18-24 months. The cause of erectile dysfunction following radiation therapy is radiation-induced trauma and damage to blood vessels, the neurovascular bundles and to the parts of the penile anatomy that are within the radiation field.

Ejaculation changes can also occur following radiation. These may include diminished or absent volume of semen, discomfort during ejaculation, blood in the ejaculate, a small amount of urine released with ejaculation and decreased intensity of orgasm.

Androgen deprivation therapy that is often combined with radiation therapy to optimize the effect of the radiation can compound the potential sexual side effects of the radiation, particularly with respect to loss of libido.

SEXUAL ISSUES AFTER ANDROGEN DEPRIVATION THERAPY

Androgen deprivation therapy results in castrate levels of testosterone with loss of libido. Although testosterone is not a necessity for achieving and maintaining erections (pre-pubertal boys obtain excellent erections, but lack libido), it certainly helps the process. Additionally, since testosterone helps sustain penile tissue health and integrity, long-term androgen deprivation therapy may result in diminished penile length and girth. Furthermore, the consequences of long-term androgen deprivation, including loss of muscle and bone mass, weight gain, hot flashes and occasional breast growth and tenderness, can negatively affect body image, masculinity, confidence and sexuality.

SEXUAL ISSUES AFTER FOCAL ABLATIVE THERAPIES

Erectile dysfunction is an expected outcome following cryosurgery. High intensity focused ultrasound uses heat to destroy prostate tissue, which can potentially damage nerves and give rise to erectile dysfunction as well as other sexual issues.

Chapter 34: What to Expect of Sexual Function with Aging

Before fully exploring prostate cancer and sexuality, a discussion of expectations of sexual function with the aging process is in order. This material is excerpted from the most popular of my over 350 weekly blogs written over the past seven years. Although much of what follows is written tongue-in-cheek, the underlying basis is entirely factual.

It is shocking how ill prepared we are for aging. We are largely uninformed about the process, so the best we can do is sit back and observe changes as they unfold. Aging can be unkind and Father Time does not spare sexual function. Although erectile dysfunction is not inevitable, with each passing decade there is an increasing prevalence of it. Present in some form in 40% of men by age 40, with each decade thereafter an additional 10% join the ED club. All aspects of sexuality decline, although sexual interest and drive suffer the least depreciation, leading to a swarm of men who are eager, but frequently unable—a most frustrating combination.

GUIDE TO SEXUAL FUNCTION BY DECADE

I have arbitrarily broken this down by decade with the understanding that these are general trends and that an individual may vary greatly from others in his age group, depending upon genetics, lifestyle, luck and other factors. There are 30-year-old men who have major sexual issues and 80-year-old men who are veritable "studs," so age per se is not the ultimate factor.

I crafted what follows after more than 30 years in the urology trenches, working the front line with thousands of patient interactions. Furthermore, I am a 60-something year-old, keenly observant of the subtle changes that I have personally witnessed, (although I must report that I am still holding my own). Educational books are available on many topics regarding expected experiences, such as "What to Expect When You're Expecting," but I have yet to see "The

171

Manual of Man," explaining the changes we might expect to experience as time goes on.

Age 18-30: Your sexual appetite is mighty and sex often occupies the front burners of your mind. It requires very little stimulation to achieve an erection—even the wind blowing the right way might be enough to stimulate a rigid, gravity-defying erection, pointing proudly at the heavens. The sight of an attractive woman, the smell of her perfume, merely the thought of her can arouse you fully. You get erections even when you don't want them... if there was only a way to bank these for later in life! You wake up in the middle of the night sporting a rigid erection. When you climax, the orgasm is intense, forceful and powerful. When you arise from sleep, it is not just you that has arisen, but also your penis.

It doesn't get better than this... you are an invincible king... a professional athlete at the pinnacle of your career! All right, maybe not invincible... you do have an Achilles heel—you may at times ejaculate rapidly because you are hyper-excitable and sometimes in a new sexual situation you may have performance anxiety, a form of stage fright brought on by your all-powerful mind dooming the capabilities of your perfectly normal plumbing.

Age 30-40: Changes occur ever so slowly, perhaps so gradually that they are barely noticeable. Your sex drive remains vigorous, but not as obsessive and all-consuming as it once was. You can still get quality erections, but they may not occur as spontaneously, as frequently and with such little provocation as they did previously. You may require some touch stimulation to develop full rigidity. You still wake up in the middle of the night with an erection and experience "morning wood." Ejaculations and orgasms are hardy, but you may notice some subtle differences, with your "rifle" being a little less powerful and of smaller caliber. The time it takes to achieve another erection after ejaculation increases. You are that athlete in the twilight of his career, seasoned and experienced, with the premature ejaculation of yonder years occurring much less frequently.

Age 40-50: After age 40, changes become more obvious. You are still interested in sex, but not nearly with the passion of two decades earlier. You can usually get a decent-quality erection, but it now often requires more tactile stimulation and the rock-star rigidity of years gone by has given way to a "firm" penis, still quite suitable for penetration. The gravity-defying erections don't have quite the upward angle they used to. At times, you may lose the erection before the sexual act is completed. You notice that orgasms have lost some of their kick and ejaculation has become feebler than previously. Getting a second erection after climax is not only more difficult, but also may be something that you no longer have much interest in. All in all though, you still have some game left.

Age 50-60: Sex is still important to you and your desire is still there but is typically diminished. Your erection is still respectable and functional, but not the majestic sight it once was, and touch is often a necessity for full arousal. Nighttime and morning erections become fewer and further between. The frequency of intercourse declines while the occurrence of losing the erection before the sexual act is complete increases. A more dribbling-quality ejaculation occurs with diminished volume and force, begging the question of why you are "drying up." Orgasms are less intense and at times it feels like nothing much happened—more "firecracker" than "fireworks." Getting a second erection is difficult, and you find much more delight in going to sleep rather than pursuing a sexual encore. Sex is no longer a sport, but a recreational activity... sometimes just reserved for the weekends.

Age 60-70: "Sexagenarian" is quite the misleading word... more apt a term for the 18-30-year-old group, because your sex life doesn't compare to theirs —they are the athletes and you the spectators. Your testosterone level has plummeted over the decades, probably accounting for your somewhat diminished desire. Erections are still obtainable with some coaxing, but they are not five-star erections, more like three stars, suitable for penetration, but not the rigid flagpoles of yonder years. They are less reliable, and at times your penis suffers with "attention deficit disorder," unable to focus and loses its mojo prematurely, unable to complete the task at hand. Spontaneous erections, nighttime, and early morning erections become rare occurrences. Climax is not so climactic and explosive ejaculations are a matter of history. At times, you think you climaxed, but are unsure because the sensation was frankly un-sensational. Ejaculation is down to a mere dribble. Seconds?...

no thank you... that is reserved for helpings on the dinner table! Sex is no longer a recreational activity, but an occasional amusement.

Age 70-80: When asked about his sexual function, my 70-something-year-old patient replied: "Retired... and I'm really upset that I'm not even upset." You may still have some lingering sexual desire left in you, but it's a far cry from the fire in your groin that you had when you were young. With physical coaxing and coercion, your penis can at times be prodded to rise to the occasion, like a cobra responding to the beck and call of the flute of the snake charmer. The quality of erections has noticeably dropped, with penile fullness without the rigidity that used to make penetration such a breeze. At times, the best that you can do is to obtain a partially inflated erection that cannot penetrate, despite pushing, shoving and manipulating. Spontaneous erections have gone the way of the 8-track player. Thank goodness for discovering that even a limp penis can be stimulated to climax, so it is still possible for you to experience sexual intimacy, although the cli-"max" is more like a cli-"min."

Age 80-90: You are now a full-fledged member of a group that has an ever-increasing constituency—the ED club. Although you as an octogenarian may still be able to have sex, most of your brethren cannot; however, they remain appreciative that at least they still have their penises to use as spigots, allowing them to stand to urinate, a distinct competitive advantage over the womenfolk. Compounding the problem is that your spouse is no longer a spring chicken and because she has likely been post-menopausal for many years, she has a significantly reduced sex drive, vaginal dryness, and perhaps medical problems that make sex downright difficult, if not impossible. If you are able to have sex on your birthday and anniversary, you are doing much better than most. To quote one of my octogenarian patients in reference to his penis: "It's like walking around with a dead fish."

Age 90-100: To quote the comedian George Burns: "Sex at age 90 is like trying to shoot pool with a rope." You are grateful to be alive and in the grand scheme of things, sex is low on the list of priorities. You can live vicariously through pleasant memories of your days of glory that are lodged deep in the recesses of your mind, as long as your memory holds out! When and if you do get an erection, you never want to waste it!

Chapter 35: An Erection is a Symphony

Erections are often taken for granted, thought of as a simple act of nature. In reality, achieving a fully rigid penis is a rather complicated physiological event. To help explain the complexity of erections, I use a symphony orchestra as a metaphor.

Achieving an erection is a "symphony" that results from the interplay of four "orchestral sections": nerves, blood vessels, erectile smooth muscle, and erectile skeletal muscle (pelvic floor muscles). The "conductor" of the orchestra is the brain (the main sex organ). Although each "musician" within the orchestral sections has a unique role, all work together harmoniously to create a beautiful "symphony." If any individual musician or orchestral section is off key, the disharmony can cause the "symphony" to be flawed, resulting in a sub-par performance.

SECTIONS OF THE ORCHESTRA

Nerves: *Think of the nerves as the string instruments (violin, viola, cello and double bass) vibrating in sync.*

The penis has a rich supply of nerves that connect with the spinal cord and brain. Without these nerves and connections, the penis would be without sensation, cut off from the rest of the body and incapable of responding to touch or erotic stimulation. The paired cavernous nerves that convey the message to the penis to fill with blood are anatomically intimate with the prostate gland.

How things work when nerves are functioning well:

- When the penis is stimulated by touch, nerves relay information to spinal cord centers, which then relay the message to the penile arteries to increase blood flow, resulting in the penis becoming engorged with blood.

- Touch to the penis is also conveyed directly to the brain, enhancing the reflex spinal cord response.

- Erotic stimulation (visual cues, sounds, smells, touch, thoughts, memories, etc.) further stimulates the penis from excitatory nerve pathways that descend from the brain.

- With touch stimulation of the head of the penis, a reflex contraction of the pelvic floor muscles occurs, which causes more blood to flow into the penis, leading to a fully rigid erection.

Blood vessels: *Think of the blood vessels as the percussion instruments (piano, xylophone, cymbals, drums, etc.) pulsing rhythmically.*

Inflation of the penis is all about blood inflow and trapping. When there are issues with the influx or trapping of blood, it becomes challenging to obtain and/or maintain an erection.

How things work when the blood vessels are functioning well:

- With touch or erotic stimulation, the cavernous nerves convey the message to the penile arteries to relax, which increases penile blood flow.

Erectile smooth muscle: *Think of the erectile smooth muscle as the woodwind instruments (piccolos, flutes, oboes, clarinets and bassoons).*

The erectile smooth muscle within the sinuses of the erectile chambers governs the inflation/deflation status of the penis. When the smooth muscle is contracted (squeezed), the penis cannot inflate with blood, but when the muscle relaxes, blood gushes into the sinuses and inflates the penis.

As we age, smooth muscle in all arteries of the body stiffens, causing high blood pressure (essential hypertension); paralleling this, there is an age-related stiffness of the erectile smooth muscle, which can cause difficulty obtaining and/or maintaining an erection.

How things work when the erectile smooth muscle is functioning well:

- With touch or erotic stimulation, the smooth muscle within the sinuses of the erectile chambers relaxes, under control of the cavernous nerves, which allows blood to flow into and fill the sinuses.

- As the sinuses approach complete filling, veins that drain them are pinched, trapping blood within the sinuses.

- This smooth muscle relaxation results in penile blood pressure becoming equal with the systolic blood pressure (normally 120 millimeters) and an engorged penis, plump but not rigid.

Erectile skeletal muscles (pelvic floor muscles): *Think of the erectile skeletal muscles as the brass instruments (trumpets, French horns, trombones, and tubas), which are capable of the loudest sounds in the orchestra. These instruments are particularly important to the most booming, powerful and exciting portions of the music, corresponding to the role of the pelvic floor muscles that maintain rigidity and drive ejaculation and climax.*

The pelvic floor muscles are the "rigidity" muscles, necessary for transforming the plump penis into a rock-hard penis. These muscles surround and compress the deep, internal roots of the penis, causing backflow of pressurized blood into the penis, responsible for obtaining and maintaining full rigidity. When the penis is erect, it is these pelvic floor muscles that are responsible for the ability to lift one's penis up and down as the muscles are contracted and relaxed. These muscles are also responsible for ejaculation—compressing the urethra rhythmically to cause the expulsion of semen.

An erection—in mechanical (hydraulic) terms—is when the penile blood inflow is maximized while outflow is minimized, resulting in an inflated and rigid penis. The pressure in the penis at the time of a fully rigid erection is greater than 200 millimeters, the only organ in the male body where high blood pressure is both acceptable and necessary for healthy function. If the systemic blood pressure was this high, it would be considered a "hypertensive crisis." As an aside, this explains why blood pressure pills are the most common medications associated with erectile dysfunction.

How things work when the pelvic floor muscles are functioning well:

179

- With touch stimulation of the head of the penis, there is a reflex contraction of the pelvic floor muscles; every time the head of the penis is stimulated, the pelvic floor muscles reflexively contract.

- The pelvic floor muscles surround the roots of the penis and as they compress and squeeze the penile roots with each contraction, blood within the roots is forced back into the external penis. This pushes more blood into the penis and causes increased clamping of venous outflow, a tourniquet-like effect resulting in penile high blood pressure and full-fledged rigidity—a brass-hard penis.

Brain: *Think of the brain as the conductor of the orchestra—the maestro—who has the vital role of unifying and coordinating the individual performers, setting the tempo, executing meter, "listening" critically and shaping the sound of the ensemble accordingly. The conductor is the key player and if he is having an off day and does not bring his "A" game, there will be disharmony in the orchestra and the symphony will be flat and unimpressive.*

Psychological and emotional factors have a significant impact on erectile function. Mood, stress, anxiety, fears, interpersonal and relationship issues, etc.—acting via the mind-body connection and mediated via the release of neurochemicals—can influence erectile function for better or worse. Stress, for example, induces the adrenal glands to release a surge of adrenaline. Adrenaline constricts blood vessels, which has a negative effect on erections, the basis for the common occurrence of adrenaline-fueled performance anxiety.

In summary, an erection is a highly complex "symphony," orchestrated by the main sex organ—the brain—and executed at the level of the penis via the individual performances of the "orchestral members" who comprise the orchestral sections—the nerves, blood vessels, erectile smooth muscle and the pelvic floor muscles. All orchestral members play a vital role in the creation of a magical synergy, resulting in a spirited, powerful, passionate performance that climaxes in a tension-releasing "symphonic finale."

Chapter 36: Use It or Lose It

Our bodies demand physical activity in order to function optimally. For example, our bones require weight bearing and a variety of movements and biomechanical stresses in order to stay well mineralized and in peak functional form. The same holds true for every organ in our body—to maintain maximal functioning they need to be put into the service for which they were designed. As much as our bodies adapt positively to resistance, so they will adapt negatively to a lack of resistance. For example, after wearing a cast on one's arm for 6 weeks, there is noticeable wasting of the arm muscles, otherwise known as "disuse atrophy." This phenomenon will occur to any body part—including the penis—not used in the manner for which it was designed.

The penis is truly a marvel of design and engineering. It is uniquely capable of increasing its blood flow by a factor of 40-50 times over baseline in a matter of nanoseconds. This is accomplished by relaxation of the smooth muscle within the arteries supplying the erectile chambers and within the erectile sinuses of the erectile chambers. This sudden rush of blood is not the case in our non-genital organs, in which blood flow can be increased upon demand (e.g., our muscles when exercising), but nowhere to the extent that it happens in the penis.

Achieving an erection not only results in a rigid penis capable of sexual penetration, but also serves to keep the penile tissues richly oxygenated, elastic and functioning well. The dramatic increase in penile blood flow that occurs with an erection enhances subsequent erectile performance via the release of nitric oxide, one of the most important chemical drivers of erections. Current theories propose that nocturnal erections achieved during the REM (rapid eye movement) phase of sleep are for the purpose of keeping penile tissues well-oxygenated and healthy.

In the absence of regular sexual activity, disuse atrophy (wasting away with a decline in structure and function) of penile smooth muscle and erectile tissues can occur. In a vicious cycle, the poor blood flow resulting from lack of use produces a state of poor oxygen levels in the penile tissues that, in turn, can induce scarring, resulting in a loss of penile length and girth and negatively affecting one's ability to achieve an erection. Herein lies the importance of getting "back in the saddle" as soon as possible following prostatectomy.

Studies have found that sexual intercourse on a regular basis protects against erectile dysfunction and that the risk of erectile dysfunction is inversely related to the frequency of intercourse. Men reporting intercourse less than once weekly have a two-fold higher incidence of erectile dysfunction as compared to men reporting intercourse once weekly.

Now for some interesting trivia:

- The spongy tissue in the erectile chambers is virtually identical to the spongy tissue in our facial sinuses. (My pathologist friend claims that he can't tell the difference under a microscope.)

- When this spongy tissue in the penis becomes congested with blood, an erection occurs; when it happens in the facial sinuses, nasal congestion (a stuffed nose) occurs.

- A side effect of oral erectile dysfunction medications (Viagra, Levitra, Cialis and Stendra) is nasal congestion... now you understand why.

- Prolonged erections (a.k.a. priapism) are often treated with the same medications used to treat nasal congestion, such as phenylephrine, which is commonly used in nasal sprays.

- The spongy tissue in the erectile chambers is surrounded by connective tissue known as the "tunica albuginea," the second toughest connective tissue in our bodies (the toughest being the "dura mater" that surrounds our brains and spinal cord).

- Many mammals have a bone in their penis ("os penis") that provides the rigidity for sexual intercourse. Humans, lacking such a bone, have evolved in such a way such that erections are hydraulic based. Blood—used for transportation of oxygen, nutrients, hormones, waste products, etc.—is employed for a different purpose, as a hydraulic fluid that is pressurized to allow rigidity. What a truly amazing feat of evolution!

Chapter 37: Practical Approach To Erectile Dysfunction

A pragmatic approach to managing ED begins with simple and sensible solutions and if unsuccessful, proceeds with more complex and involved strategies. This chapter is an overview of treatment options with a more detailed discussion of the individual options in the chapters that follow. This chapter is appropriate to any man with ED issues, not only those men with problems following treatment of prostate cancer.

A practical approach to ED—similar to the strategy for most medical issues—entails a history, physical examination and basic laboratory tests, with more extensive testing used on a tailored and individualized basis. If the initial evaluation indicates a high likelihood that the ED is psychological or emotional in origin, referral to a qualified psychologist, psychiatrist or sexual counselor is in order. If the lab evaluation is indicative of low testosterone, additional hormone tests to determine the precise cause of the low testosterone need to be done prior to consideration for treatment aimed at normalizing the testosterone level. If testing shows unrecognized or poorly controlled diabetes or a risky lipid and cholesterol profile, appropriate medical referral is vital.

ED can oftentimes be a "canary in the trousers"—an indicator that a more pervasive underlying medical problem exists. In other words, erection quality can serve as a barometer of cardiovascular health, with the presence of rigid and durable erections a gauge of overall good cardiovascular health and the presence of ED a clue to poor cardiovascular health. Since the penile arteries are generally small (diameter 1-2 millimeters) and the coronary arteries larger (4 millimeters), it stands to reason that if blood vessel disease is affecting the tiny penile arteries, it may affect the larger coronary arteries as well—if not now, then at some time in the near future. For this reason, men with ED should undergo a basic medical evaluation seeking arterial disease elsewhere in the body.

Although a nuanced and individualized approach is always desirable, four general lines of treatment for ED are defined—from simple to complex—in an analogous way that tiers of treatment can be considered for other common medical issues such as degenerative joint disease.

FOUR TIER TREATMENT OF ERECTILE DYSFUNCTION

First-line: Lifestyle makeover

A healthy lifestyle can "reverse" ED naturally, as opposed to "managing" it. Since ED can often be considered a "chronic disease," healthy lifestyle choices can reverse it, prevent its progression and even prevent its onset.

Since sexual functioning is based upon many body components working harmoniously (central and peripheral nerve system, hormone system, blood vessel system, smooth and skeletal muscles), the first-line approach is to nurture every cell, tissue and organ in the body. This translates to achieving "fighting" weight, adopting a heart-healthy and penis-healthy diet (whole foods, nutrient-dense, calorie-light, avoiding processed and refined junk foods), exercising, getting adequate quantity and quality of sleep, stopping use of tobacco, consuming alcohol in moderation, and stress reduction (yoga, meditation, massage, hot baths, etc.). Aside from general exercises (cardiovascular, core, strength and flexibility training), specific pelvic floor muscle exercises ("man-Kegels") are beneficial to improve the strength, power and endurance of the penile "rigidity" muscles. More about pelvic floor muscle training in the chapter that follows.

If a healthy lifestyle can be adopted, sexual function will often improve dramatically, in parallel to overall health improvements. Since many medications have side effects that negatively impact sexual function, a bonus of lifestyle improvement is potentially needing lower dosages or perhaps eliminating medications (blood pressure, cholesterol, diabetic meds, etc.), which can result in further improving sexual function.

"The food you eat is so profoundly instrumental to your health that breakfast, lunch and dinner are in fact exercises in medical decision making."
—Thomas Campbell, MD

Second-line: ED pills and mechanical devices

It is my opinion that the oral ED medications should be reserved for when lifestyle optimization fails to improve the sexual issues. This may be at odds with some physicians who find it convenient to simply prescribe meds, and with some patients who want a quick and easy fix. However, as good as Viagra, Levitra, Cialis and Stendra may be, they are expensive, have side effects, are not effective for every patient and cannot be used in everyone, as there are medical situations and certain medications that may preclude their use. The exception to reserving ED meds for non-responders to lifestyle improvement is for men after prostatectomy or other treatments for prostate cancer who have ED and need to be on a penile rehabilitation program (more about this in the chapter on erection recovery).

In the second-line category, I also include the mechanical, non-pharmacological, non-surgical devices, including the vacuum suction, vibration, and penile traction devices. Even though it is not yet FDA approved, I also place low-intensity penile shockwave therapy in this category.

Vacuum erection devices are mechanical means of producing an erection in which the penis is placed within a plastic cylinder that is connected to a manual or battery-powered vacuum. Negative pressure engorges the penis with blood and a constriction band is temporarily placed around the base of the penis to maintain the erection. 80% of men can achieve good rigidity, but many do not continue using the device because of its cumbersome nature.

Venous constriction devices are used in conjunction with the vacuum erection devices to trap blood in the penis and help maintain the erection. They also can be used without the suction devices in certain circumstances. Men who find these beneficial are usually able to obtain a reasonable quality rigid erection but tend to lose it prematurely.

Vibration devices were traditionally employed to provoke ejaculation in men with spinal cord injuries who desired to father children. Subsequently, they have achieved broader utility and are now also used to facilitate erections in men with ED. Dual-armed vibratory stimulation of the penile shaft is capable of inducing an erection and ultimately ejaculation.

Penile traction devices use mechanical pulling forces to lengthen and/or straighten the penis to manage or prevent penile shortening and angulation.

Low-intensity shockwave therapy is an exciting new treatment option that uses acoustic energy to cause mechanical stress and microtrauma to erectile tissues. This stimulates the growth of new blood vessels and nerve fibers and potentially enables penile tissue to regain the ability for spontaneous erection.

Third-line: Vasodilator urethral suppositories and penile injections

These are suppositories and injections that increase penile blood flow and induce erections.

M.U.S.E. (Medical urethral system for erection) is a small medicated vasodilator pellet available in a variety of different dosages that is placed within the urinary channel of the penis after urinating. Absorption occurs through the urethra into the adjacent erectile chambers, inducing increased penile blood flow and potentially an erection. About 40% of men can achieve rigidity, but it is often inconsistent.

Prostaglandin E1 (Caverject and Edex) is injected directly into one of the erectile chambers of the penis, resulting in increased blood flow and erectile rigidity. After being taught the technique of self-injection, vasodilator medications can be used on demand, resulting in rigid and durable erections. A combination of medications can be used for optimal results—one such popularly used combination consists of papaverine, phentolamine and alprostadil, known as "Trimix." 90% or so of men achieve an excellent response, although many men are reluctant to put a needle into their penis.

Fourth-line: Penile prostheses

Penile prostheses can be life changers for men who cannot achieve a sustainable erection. Surgically implanted under anesthesia on an outpatient basis, they provide the necessary penile rigidity to have intercourse whenever and for however long desirable.

The semi-rigid device is a simple one-piece flexible rod, one of which is implanted within each of the paired erectile chambers. The penis is bent up for sexual intercourse and down for concealment. The inflatable device is a three-piece unit that is capable of inflation and deflation. Inflatable inner tubes are implanted within the erectile chambers, a fluid reservoir is implanted behind the pubic bone or abdominal muscles and a control pump in the scrotum, adjacent to the testes. When the patient desires an erection, he pumps the control pump several times, which transfers fluid from the reservoir to the inflatable inner tubes, creating a hydraulic erection that can be used for as long as desired. When the sexual act is completed, the device is deflated via the control pump, transferring fluid back to the reservoir and restoring a flaccid state.

Chapter 38: Pelvic Floor Muscle (PFM) Training: Strengthening the Little Muscles That Could

Limber hip rotators,

A powerful cardio-core,

But forget not

The oft-neglected pelvic floor

Recall that an erection occurs because of penile inflow of blood and trapping of penile outflow. Once blood inflates the erectile chambers, closure of penile veins traps the blood in the penis. At this point the penis is tumescent—plump—but not rigid. Several of the PFM engage to act as a "muscular tourniquet" that further restrict the exit of blood and with each contraction of these specialized muscles, a surge of blood flows into the erectile chambers, causing penile high blood pressure and bone-like erectile rigidity.

The outer half of the penis is exposed and the inner half is internal. The internal parts lie under the surface and are known as the penile roots. Like the roots of a tree responsible for foundational support of the trunk, branches and leaves, the roots of the penis stabilize and support the erect penis so that it stays rigid and skyward-angling and maintains an excellent "posture." The penis requires this sturdy foundational support not only to morph into a rigid erection, but also to maintain rigid stability despite exposure to the "elements"—the substantial forces associated with sexual activity—that can torque and buckle the penis. Without functional penile roots, the penis would remain limp, dangling in accordance with gravity and with a slouching posture at best.

The penile roots are enveloped by two of the superficial PFM, the ischiocavernosus (IC) and the bulbocavernosus (BC). The IC is the "erector muscle" and the BC the "ejaculator muscle." IC muscle contractions compress the penile roots to maximize and maintain erectile rigidity. Rhythmic BC muscle contractions at the time of sexual climax compress the urethra and cause the ejaculation of semen. The BC and IC muscles are also responsible for the ability to lift one's erect penis up and down (wag the penis) as they are contracted and relaxed. Although not external muscles of "glamour," they are certainly the muscles of "amour."

The PFM—although unseen and behind-the-scenes, hidden from view, and often unrecognized and misunderstood—have vital functions in addition to erection and ejaculation. They straddle the gamut of being critical for what may be considered the most pleasurable and refined of human pursuits— sex (superficial PFM)—but equally integral to what may be considered the basest of human activities—bladder and bowel function (deep PFM). The deep PFM strongly contribute to the sphincter function of the bladder and the bowel. As part of the core group of muscles, their structure and function also affect body posture, the lower back and the hips.

When the PFM are not functioning optimally, one loses the potential for full erectile rigidity, among other pelvic issues. Like other skeletal muscles, they can undergo "disuse atrophy," becoming thinner, flabbier and less functional with aging, weight gain, sedentary lifestyles, poor posture, chronic straining and other forms of trauma, including pelvic surgery (e.g., prostatectomy) and pelvic radiation. Like other skeletal muscles, positive adaptive changes can be made to them if they are trained properly. Because they are critical to healthy sexual function, exercising them can enhance sexual health, maintain sexual health, help prevent the occurrence of ED in the future and help manage ED. Specifically, pelvic floor exercises can be beneficial with respect to the following spectrum of issues: ED, ejaculation issues including premature ejaculation, stress urinary incontinence, overactive bladder, post-void dribbling and bowel urgency and incontinence.

One of the challenges of pelvic floor training is that most men do not know where their PFM are located, what they do, how to exercise them, and what benefits training these muscles may confer. In fact, many men don't even know that they have PFM. Because they are out of sight, they are often out of mind and not considered when it comes to exercise and fitness. However, although concealed from view, they deserve serious respect as they are responsible for vital functions that can be enhanced when intensified by training.

PFM training initiated before and continued after prostate cancer surgery can facilitate the resumption of both urinary control and sexual function. As the most expedient means of achieving pelvic strengthening, I highly recommend the following exercise program: PelvicRx (www.PelvicRx.com). It is a well-designed and easy to use, follow-along, interactive 4-week pelvic training DVD that offers strengthening and endurance pelvic floor exercises. It provides education, guidance, training, and feedback to confirm the engagement of the proper muscles. It is structured so that repetitions, contraction intensity and contraction duration are gradually increased over the course of the program. This progression is the key to optimizing pelvic strength and endurance.

(Disclaimer: I am co-creator of the PelvicRx program. I helped design this program because I recognized the importance for men to be properly instructed to train their PFM to optimize their urinary and sexual health following prostate cancer treatment, among other reasons.)

The reader is also referred to a book I wrote on the topic of male pelvic floor training: *MALE PELVIC FITNESS: Optimizing Sexual and Urinary Health*, published in 2014 (www.MalePelvicFitness.com).

Chapter 39: Oral Erectile Dysfunction (ED) Medications

Chemistry of penile rigidity

In an erotic situation, the cavernous nerves (extensions of the neurovascular bundles that provide the nerve input to the erectile chambers) release nitric oxide that then cause the release of the chemical messenger cGMP (cyclic guanosine monophosphate). The cGMP release causes penile smooth muscle relaxation resulting in blood flooding into the erectile chambers. As the erection gets fuller, penile veins become compressed, limiting the exit of blood and ultimately the pelvic floor muscles engage to generate maximal erectile rigidity.

Chemistry of penile flaccidity

After ejaculation, the enzyme PDE-5 (phosphodiesterase-5) is released, which causes decreased levels of cGMP, resulting in a loss of the erection and a return to the flaccid state.

ED meds

The oral ED medications include sildenafil (Viagra), tadalafil (Cialis), vardenafil (Levitra) and avanafil (Stendra). They work by inhibiting the chemical mediator of flaccidity and are known as PDE-5 inhibitors. They can be a simple and discreet solution to ED. They are taken by mouth and require anywhere from 15-60 minutes to start working. Because their absorption can be slowed by a meal, they are generally best taken on an empty stomach to optimize their absorption. Although they can result in some increase in penile fullness (tumescence) without sexual stimulation, sexual stimulation is a must in order to induce a fully rigid erection.

The arrival of this class of medication in 1998 revolutionized the management of ED. Although each of the available medications in this class is effective in improving erection issues for most men, there are subtle differences among the four that provide potential advantages and disadvantages. Trial and error may be required to determine which works best for an individual's needs.

Although effective for many men, they will not work for everyone. If there is significant nerve or blood vessel compromise to the penis, they will likely be ineffective. It is important to know that the same ED drug at the same dose may work variably depending on the particular time and situation, sometimes more effectively than at other times since there are so many factors that determine erectile rigidity.

Men who are taking any of the nitrate class of drugs (cardiac medications of the nitroglycerine family that are used for angina) should never use the oral ED meds or serious consequences may result, including a dramatic drop in blood pressure. (Perhaps you might remember Jack Nicholson's situation in the movie *Something's Gotta Give?*).

Viagra This was the first of the group, released in 1998. Dosed at 25, 50 or 100 mg, the half-life (the period of time required for its concentration in the blood to be reduced by one-half) is about 4 hours. It is taken on demand with an onset of 15-60 minutes and remains active for 12 or so hours.

Viagra trivia: Viagra was discovered by chance. Pfizer scientists, in an effort to find a new drug to treat high blood pressure and chest pain, conducted a clinical trial with this experimental medicine that works by causing blood vessels to dilate. The medication did not work particularly well for the intended purposes of the study but had a side effect in that it dramatically improved erections. When the study ended, the participants were profoundly disturbed that the drug was no longer available. The rest is history.

More Viagra trivia: The name Viagra was born as a fusion of the word "vigor" (physical strength) and "Niagara" (the most powerful waterfall in North America).

Even more Viagra trivia: Viagra is not only used for ED. A 20 mg dose is effective for children with pulmonary hypertension, a condition in which the blood vessels in the lungs have abnormally high blood pressures.

The most common side effects of Viagra are headache, facial flushing, upset stomach, and nasal and sinus congestion. Less frequent side effects are temporary changes in color vision, sensitivity to light and blurry vision.

Levitra This drug came to market in 2003, available in 10 mg and 20 mg doses. The effectiveness and side effect profiles are similar to Viagra; however, there are no reports of visual distortions as side effects. It is taken on demand and has an onset of 15-60 minutes and a half-life of about 4 hours, remaining active for 12 or so hours.

Levitra trivia: The name Levitra derives from "elevate"; in French "le" indicates masculinity and "vitra" suggests vitality.

More Levitra trivia: Levitra is also formulated in a minty, dissolves-in-your-mouth 10 mg formulation called Staxyn. Staxyn dissolves on the tongue and is absorbed directly through the oral mucosa, so slower absorption because of taking the medication at the time of a meal is not an issue.

Cialis FDA approved in 2003, it is available in 2.5, 5, 10 and 20 mg doses. The effectiveness and side effect profiles are similar to Viagra. Uniquely, Cialis has a long duration of action that has earned it the nickname "the weekender" as it can be taken on Friday evening and remain effective for the rest of the weekend without the need for an additional dose. This affords a considerable advantage in terms of spontaneity. Cialis is either taken on demand (usually 10 or 20 mg, although 5 mg can be effective as well) or on a daily basis (2.5 or 5 mg) and has an onset of 15-60 minutes and remains active for 36 or so hours.

Cialis trivia: Cialis is also approved to treat children with pulmonary hypertension.

In 2012, daily Cialis (2.5 and 5 mg) was FDA approved for the management of urinary symptoms due to benign prostate enlargement.

Cialis can occasionally cause backaches and other muscle aches. Cialis is not affected by eating fatty meals, which can slow the absorption of the alternative ED meds (with the exception of Staxyn).

Stendra FDA approved in 2012, it is available in 50, 100 and 200 mg doses. It has the advantage of a rapid onset of action. It is taken on demand and has an onset of about 15 minutes and remains active for 12 or so hours.

Stendra trivia: The name Stendra probably is a derivative of the word "extends."

Recommendations to improve effectiveness of the oral ED medications

1. Take on an empty stomach or after a low-fat meal.

2. Take 45-60 minutes before anticipated sexual activity.

3. Ensure sexual stimulation since they are ineffective without.

4. Increase to a higher dose if initial dose is ineffective.

5. Using daily dosing as opposed to on-demand may improve effectiveness.

6. Continue to use periodically even if ineffective initially because of expected gradual improvement in erections after prostate treatment.

My take

Viagra 100 mg is the most potent of the group, but will also incur the most side effects, particularly facial flushing and potentially a nasty headache. Levitra is very similar in most respects to Viagra in terms of effectiveness and side effects. Rarely, Viagra can cause an alteration in color perception. Cialis is overall the best of the bunch because of its long duration, the spontaneity factor, the ability to take it with a fatty meal and its dual utility of helping urination as well as sexual function. The downside to Cialis is occasional muscle aches. The rapid onset of Stendra confers a small advantage.

Many men are capable of functioning satisfactorily without any of these medications but find that taking a "recreational" (low dose) enhances erectile capability and takes years off the functional age of the penis. It is particularly useful for those with performance anxiety.

Many men who undergo nerve-sparing prostatectomy or image-guided radiation therapy will be able to have good quality erections with the use of oral meds. It is common practice after prostatectomy to start daily Cialis 5 mg or alternative ED medications to accelerate the erection recovery process. (More about this in the chapter on erection recovery.)

Chapter 40: Vacuum Erection Device (VED)

The VED, a.k.a. penis pump, is one of the oldest treatments for erectile dysfunction. It is a mechanical means of inducing an erection that does not utilize medications or surgery. It works by creating negative pressures that cause an influx of blood into the erectile chambers, resulting in penile expansion and erection. It is an effective means of inducing a penile erection suitable for sexual intercourse—even in difficult-to-treat men who have diabetes, spinal cord injury, or after prostatectomy. The device is also useful in the post-operative period following prostatectomy to maintain penile length, girth and tissue integrity. It can also be used prior to penile prosthesis surgery in order to enhance penile length and facilitate the placement of the largest possible implant.

"Tissue expansion" occurs in response to forces that can be internal or external. Internal tissue expansion occurs naturally with pregnancy, weight gain and the presence of slow growing tumors. Plastic surgeons commonly tap into the tissue expansion principle by using implantable expanders prior to breast reconstructive surgery. The VED is a form of external tissue expansion that uses negative pressures applied to the penis to stretch the tissues of the penile erectile chambers. The resultant influx of blood increases tissue oxygenation, activates tissue nutrient factors, mobilizes stem cells, helps prevent tissue scarring and induces an erection. It is thus advantageous in the preservation and restoration of penile anatomy and function.

There are many commercially available devices on the market, which share in common a cylinder chamber with one end closed off, a vacuum pump and a constriction ring. The penis is inserted into the cylinder chamber and an erection is induced by virtue of a vacuum that creates negative pressures and sucks blood into the erectile chambers of the penis. To maintain the erection after the vacuum is released, a constriction ring is applied to the base of the penis. The end result is a rigid penis capable of penetrative intercourse.

The VED is prepared by placing a constriction ring over the open end of the cylinder. A water-soluble lubricant is applied to the base of the penis to achieve a tight seal when the penis is placed into the cylinder. Either a manual or automatic pump is used to generate negative pressures within the cylinder, which pulls blood into the penis, causing fullness and ultimately rigidity. Once full rigidity is achieved, the constriction ring is pushed off the cylinder onto the base of the penis and the penis removed from the cylinder.

A distinct advantage of the VED is that it is a simple mechanical treatment that does not require drugs or surgery. It can be used to enhance the speed and extent of sexual recovery after prostatectomy, minimize the decrease in penile length and girth that may occur, and enable achievement of a rigid erection suitable for sexual intercourse. Clinical studies have clearly demonstrated that VED use after prostatectomy helps preserve existing penile length and prevents loss of length.

Disadvantages are the cumbersome nature of the preparation process and the need for preparation time, which significantly impairs spontaneity. Another disadvantage is the need for wearing the constriction device, which can be uncomfortable and cause "hinging" at the site of application of the constriction ring resulting in a floppy penis (because of lack of rigidity of the deep roots of the penis) as well as impairing ejaculation. Other potential issues are discomfort and pain, coolness, numbness, altered sensation, engorgement of the penile head and bruising. Importantly, the ring should never be left on for more than 30 minutes to minimize the likelihood of problems. After the sexual act is completed, the constriction ring must be removed. Although effective even in difficult-to-treat populations, many discontinue using the device because of its unwieldy nature and the preparation and time involved. Despite the disadvantages, the VED can be a useful tool in the penile rehabilitation process. More about this in the chapter on erection recovery.

Note: For a nice selection of VEDs, visit the Urology Health Store: www.UrologyHealthStore.com

Chapter 41: Venous Constriction Devices

Venous constriction devices are bands that are placed around the base of the penis or sometimes around the base of the penis and scrotum to maintain erectile rigidity. These constriction bands are particularly useful in men who can obtain rigidity but prematurely lose the erection, which is often due to "corporal-venous occlusive dysfunction," a.k.a. venous leak, in which there is insufficient trapping of blood.

Constriction devices provide compression around the circumference of the penis to help prevent volume and pressure loss from the engorged erectile chambers, providing more sustained erections. They should never be left on for longer than 30 minutes to minimize the likelihood of serious potential problems due to the effect of the band on the blood supply to the penis. In addition to their utility in helping maintain erectile rigidity, they are also useful for men who leak urine during foreplay, sexual intercourse or climax. There are many varieties available that go under different names including bands, loops, lassos, ties and rings. The sex toy industry refers to venous constriction devices as "cock rings."

Note: For a nice selection of venous constriction devices, visit the Urology Health Store: www.UrologyHealthStore.com

Chapter 42: Penile Vibration Stimulation

For many years, vibration devices in men were predominantly used for spinal cord injured patients who desired to father children but were prevented from doing so because of inability to ejaculate resulting from the neurological injury. When vibration stimulation is applied to the head of the penis of a spinal cord injury patient, a reflex erection is initiated and ultimately ejaculation will occur, a means of collecting semen in order to perform insemination.

Recent years have witnessed expansion of the use of vibration devices to the non-spinal cord injured population suffering with ED and ejaculation issues. Like the vacuum erection device, they offer a non-pharmacological, non-surgical option to the management of sexual dysfunction for men. Medical-grade penile vibratory stimulation units are specifically designed for male anatomy, consisting of dual vibration heads for the purpose of providing stimulation to both the upper and lower surfaces of the penis. Penile vibration stimulation is one of the many options available for the prostatectomy patient to help expedite return of erectile function.

Note: For a nice selection of penile vibration stimulation devices, visit the Urology Health Store: www.UrologyHealthStore.com

204

Chapter 43: Penile Traction Therapy

Tissue expansion is a commonly employed technique used by plastic and reconstructive surgeons to expand specific anatomical parts. "Traction therapy," a.k.a. "mechanical transduction," is the application of forces that pull on tissues in order to expand them. Traction ultimately leads to cellular proliferation and formation of new collagen (the main structural protein found in connective tissue).

Successful tissue expansion requires application of a sufficient pulling force and adequate time of exposure to the force. When so applied to body parts for extended periods of time, mechanical forces and stresses are capable of positively affecting cellular and tissue growth, resulting in gradual lengthening and expansion.

Traction therapy can be applied to the penis to manage or prevent penile shortening and angulation. By using mechanical pulling forces, traction is capable of lengthening and/or straightening the penis. Penile traction therapy can be used for management of penile shortening following treatment for prostate cancer, as a management of Peyronie's disease and prior to penile prosthesis implant surgery to optimize penile length.

An advantage of traction therapy is its relatively noninvasive nature. Disadvantages include the cumbersome nature of wearing the device and the relatively long treatment period required (several hours daily for months) for effective penile lengthening.

Note: For a high quality penile traction device, visit the Urology Health Store: www.UrologyHealthStore.com

Chapter 44: Low Intensity Penile Shockwave Therapy

For many years, urologists have used focused shockwave therapy to pulverize kidney stones, revolutionizing their treatment. A much tamer form of shockwaves–low intensity shockwave therapy—is a novel treatment for ED. Acoustic vibrations when applied to the penis cause cellular micro-trauma and mechanical stress that stimulates the growth of new blood vessels and nerve fibers and induces structural changes and adaptive pathways that can regenerate and remodel damaged erectile tissues. The end result is improved penile blood flow and erectile function. In addition to its application for ED, it is also being used for the management of Peyronie's disease.

Shockwave therapy uniquely modifies ED by improving the health of the erectile tissues. This is unlike most traditional ED treatments that do not treat the underlying cause of the problem and essentially function as "Band-Aids." Although not yet FDA approved in the United States, clinical trials have shown both subjective improvement in erection quality as well as objective increased penile blood flow and erectile rigidity. Treatment variables include the shockwave power setting, number of shocks delivered, the precise sites treated and duration of the treatment. The procedure is well tolerated aside from a slight pricking or vibrating sensation that is perceived during the delivery of the shockwaves. Further clinical investigation is necessary to determine optimal treatment protocols. It is highly likely that in the near future it will be approved by the FDA.

Chapter 45: Medicated Urethral Suppositories

MUSE (medicated urethral system for erection) is a vasodilating drug formulated as a urethral suppository that can increase penile blood flow and induce an erection. MUSE consists of prostaglandin E1 (Alprostadil) pellets—available in 125, 250, 500, and 1000 microgram dosages—that are placed into the urinary channel after urinating. Absorption occurs through the urethra into the adjacent erectile chambers.

A fundamental problem with MUSE is that it is placed in the urethra, which has little to no role in erectile function. While the urethra is surrounded by one of the erectile chambers (spongy body) that becomes plump, it does not become rigid at the time of an erection. The neighboring erectile chambers (cavernous bodies) are the paired structures that are responsible for erectile rigidity. MUSE relies on the medication being locally absorbed by the spongy body and then diffusing into the adjacent cavernous bodies. The onset of MUSE is 15 minutes or so, and when effective, which it is in only 30-40% of men, the erection will last for about one hour.

Why did Willie Sutton rob banks? Because that's where the money is. When it comes to erections, the money is the cavernous bodies. Using MUSE is like robbing the building next to the bank. Because it relies on absorption to adjacent structures, the dosage required is significantly higher than when the medication is injected directly into the cavernous bodies (penile injection therapy). A 1000 microgram pellet may be needed when placed within the urethra as opposed to only 10 micrograms when injected, indicative of the efficiency of injecting the medication directly into the cavernous bodies as opposed to the inefficiency of relying on absorption from the spongy body.

An applicator delivers the medicated pellet into the tip of the penis. It should be inserted after urinating, which functions to lubricate the urethra and make the administration easier. The pellet is formulated to dissolve in the small amount of urine remaining in the urethra after urination. Side effects include pain during insertion, urethral burning, aching in the penis, testicles, perineum and legs, redness of the penis and minor urethral bleeding or spotting.

My take is that although MUSE sounds reasonable in theory, in practice it is an uncomfortable means of administration and does not work particularly well. Although initially promising when first available, experience has demonstrated that most men do not find it to be a successful means of restoring erections.

Chapter 46: Penile Injection Therapy ("A Small Prick for A Bigger One")

In 1982, French vascular surgeon Dr. Ronald Virag discovered the effect on erections of the anti-spasmodic medication papaverine, which is used to relax and expand blood vessels. When he mistakenly infused this drug into the penis, thinking he was administering saline, his patient immediately developed an erection and Dr. Virag realized that a novel treatment for ED was possible.

The following year at the American Urological Association meeting in Las Vegas an event occurred that forevermore changed the treatment of ED. Giles Brindley, a British physiologist, appeared from behind the podium at the plenary session and dropped his pants in front of a large audience of urologists, unveiling his erect penis. Minutes before, he had injected a vasodilator medication (a drug that promotes penile blood inflow) into his penis. Commented one authority: *Farther down the Strip, Seigfried and Roy were making a white Bengal tiger disappear, and two circus aerialists—one sitting on the other's shoulders—were traversing a tightrope without a net. But even in Vegas they'd never seen a show like this.* Few medical developments have had the dramatic effect that Brindley's demonstration had, supporting the principle that an erection is caused by smooth muscle relaxation of the tissues of the penile erectile chambers.

Penile injections of vasodilator drugs are beneficial for a wide range of medical conditions that cause ED: psychological, neurological and hormonal causes and in men with some degree of blood vessel disease due to blocked arterial inflow. Vasodilator drugs injected directly into the penile erectile chambers bypass psychological, neurological and hormonal factors and act locally on the erectile sinus tissues, causing blood to pour into the erectile chambers, inducing a rigid erection on demand. These injectable medications can uniquely initiate an erection without sexual stimulation, as opposed to the oral ED medications that require sexual stimulation to work effectively.

A tiny needle is used to inject the vasodilator medication directly into one of the paired penile erectile chambers on one side of the penis. An erection usually occurs within 5-30 minutes and lasts for a variable amount of time, depending on the dosage used. An injection-induced erection does not interfere with one's ability to ejaculate or experience a climax. The erection will persist even after ejaculation has occurred, until the medication is out of the system.

Prostaglandin E1, a.k.a. alprostadil (Caverject, Edex) is a commonly prescribed vasodilator. Injections of this can be painful since prostaglandin is a chemical that can induce pain. Combinations of vasodilator medications are often used to obtain optimal results and induce less pain than prostaglandin E1 alone. "Bimix" consists of a combination of two vasodilators: papaverine and phentolamine. "Trimix" is a highly effective mixture of three vasodilator drugs in combination: prostaglandin E1, papaverine and phentolamine. "Quadramix" consists of four medications in combination, Trimix with atropine added. The use of combined medications increases the chances that the injection therapy will be successful.

Patients who are interested in penile injection therapy are taught the procedure during a urological office visit, at which time a test dose is administered. It is not a difficult technique to learn, although it does require dexterity. With practice and experience, one rapidly can become skilled in the process. After learning the technique, the medication can be self-administered on demand. It often requires some trial and error to get the dosage calibrated so that the erection lasts an appropriate amount of time, in accordance with individual desires.

Side effects may be pain, bleeding, bruising, scarring and prolonged erections. The most common side effect is a dull ache that is usually mild and tolerable. Again, this typically happens with prostaglandin E1 more commonly than with combinations of vasodilators. A bruise may occur at the injection site and is best prevented by applying compression on the injection site for several minutes following the injection. Occasionally, a small lump can develop at the site of repeated injections and rarely penile scarring may be a consequence.

On occasion, a prolonged erection may occur. An erection that lasts for more than four hours is a potentially serious issue that needs to be addressed. If this happens, the following may prove helpful: increasing physical activity, e.g., running up a few flights of stairs to promote a "steal" of blood from the genitals to the muscles; applying an icepack to the penis; and pseudoephedrine (Sudafed) 30-60 mg. If the erection fails to subside, it often requires the injection of a medication to reverse the effects of the vasodilator drug. This is usually done in the emergency room with cardiac monitoring.

Fact: Sadly, there are some unscrupulous medical groups who prey on unsuspecting and vulnerable ED patients, often offering injection therapy without discussion of alternative treatments and charging patients exorbitant fees for medications such as Trimix. The reality is that medications such as Trimix can be obtained at reputable compounding pharmacies via prescription from your urologist for very reasonable fees. It should not cost an arm and a leg to obtain a rigid penis!

Technique of penile injection

Preliminary tips:

- Shave the base of the penis to make the process easier.

- If possible, immediately before injecting, massage the penis to obtain some penile blood flow and filling. The injection will be easier with a fuller penis.

- Avoid superficial veins when doing the injection.

- Only one side needs to be injected even though there are two erection chambers, since they communicate.

- Hold pressure on the injection site for several minutes after the injection to avoid bleeding and bruising.

- Vary the injection site on the side that you are using to avoid scarring.

1. If you are right-handed, use your left thumb to protect the 12 o'clock position (penile nerves) and your left index finger to protect the 6 o'clock position (urethra). If you are left-handed, use your right thumb to pro-

tect the 12 o'clock position (penile nerves) and your right index finger to protect the 6 o'clock position (urethra).

2. Use an alcohol swab to cleanse the base of the penis in order to prevent infections and then set aside the swab.

3. Holding the syringe like a pen, in dart-like fashion penetrate the skin of the penis at a right angle, passing the needle as far as it will go. The site should be between the 1 o'clock and 3 o'clock position for a righty and 9 o'clock and 11 o'clock position for a lefty. The base of the shaft is the easiest location for the injection; however, because the erectile chambers run all the way to the head of the penis, any shaft location is acceptable for the injection site.

4. Inject the full contents of the syringe by applying pressure to the plunger.

5. Remove the syringe and use the alcohol swab to apply pressure to the injection site for several minutes.

6. Observe your penis becoming increasingly rigid and voilà, the rest is up to you!

Penile injection therapy—although sometimes a hard sell (pardon the pun) because of the concept of needle in penis—can be a highly effective technique for men with ED following treatment of prostate cancer. Not only does it permit achievement of a rigid erection effective for sexual intercourse, but it also helps rehabilitate the penis to maintain blood flow and tissue integrity that can be compromised in the absence of erections. More about this in the chapter on erection recovery.

Chapter 47: Penile Prostheses

Penile prostheses are highly effective means of restoring erectile function for men who do not respond to simpler measures. In many ways, penile prostheses are as quality-of-life-restoring as are total joint replacements to those suffering with arthritis, converting penile "cripples" into functional males with restored erections and resolution of the psychological and emotional anguish resulting from the loss of virility and vitality.

Since the penile prosthesis first became available over forty years ago, numerous refinements, modifications and innovations have been made. The current iterations are sophisticated and well-engineered devices composed of medical-grade synthetic materials. They are surgically implanted under anesthesia, typically on an outpatient basis. They are totally internal, with no visible external parts and function to provide sufficient penile rigidity to permit vaginal penetration. For the right man under the appropriate circumstances, the penile prosthesis can be a life changer.

Penile sensitivity, sex drive and ability to ejaculate are essentially unchanged following implantation of a penile prosthesis. Unlike a normal erection, a penile prosthesis does not result in swelling of the head of the penis nor the erectile tissue surrounding the urethra. Nonetheless, it results in a penetrable and durable erection that can restore sexual function in a man who is incapable of achieving an erection.

There are two types: semi-rigid and inflatable. I liken the difference between these two implants to the distinction between a Volkswagen and Mercedes, both effective and functional, but the latter with many more "bells and whistles." In either case, the dimensions of one's erectile chambers are precisely measured in order to size the implant properly, similar to measuring the length and width of your feet in order to ensure a good shoe fit.

A semi-rigid penile prosthesis (a.k.a. malleable implant) is a "static" implant that always remains rigid, not unlike the penile bone present in many primates, except that it can be hinged. It is bent upwards for sexual use and downwards for concealment. It consists of two malleable cylinders that are implanted within the paired penile erectile chambers through a small incision. Its advantage is its simplicity, the fact that it is less expensive than an inflatable device and its utility for patients with dexterity issues and for those with a limited reach. Its disadvantage is that it cannot go from an inflated state to a deflated state as can the inflatable penile implant, thus creating potential concealment issues. Furthermore, by virtue of the constant pressure of the implant on the soft tissues of the penis, it can be more uncomfortable than the inflatable variety and has the potential for thinning the penile flesh.

The inflatable penile prosthesis is a "dynamic" hydraulic implant designed to mimic the characteristics of a normal erection. It can be inflated and deflated at will by virtue of a self-contained hydraulic system. Cylinders (inner tubes) are implanted within the paired erectile chambers. The control pump is implanted in an accessible area of the scrotum. The third element is the reservoir that contains the fluid necessary for inflation, which is typically implanted behind the pubic bone or the abdominal wall. Tubing connects the control pump to the cylinders and to the reservoir.

When an erection is desired, the scrotal control pump is repeatedly squeezed, which transfers saline from the reservoir into the penile cylinders. As the cylinders fill, an erection develops and with each consecutive squeeze, more fluid fills the cylinders, creating a more rigid erection of wider girth. The erection will remain until the release bar located at the upper aspect of the control pump is activated. After the completion of sexual intercourse, by pressing this release bar, the fluid in the cylinders returns to the reservoir where it is again stored, returning the penis to its flaccid state. Some inflatable implants are designed to increase in girth only, whereas others increase in length and girth.

Advantages of the inflatable implant are its ability to inflate and deflate, mimicking normal erectile function and creating no issues with concealment. The penis can be kept rigid for as long as desired and will not deflate after ejaculation, unlike the flaccidity that occurs after ejaculation under normal circumstances. Disadvantages include its additional expense (although it is usually covered by insurance), the fact that it requires some degree of manual dexterity to operate, and the fact that it is more susceptible to mechanical malfunction than the semi-rigid variety because of its complexity.

Both semi-rigid and inflatable varieties of prostheses can be highly beneficial in men with ED following treatment for prostate cancer who have not responded to simpler measures.

Chapter 48: Erection Recovery: Penile Rehabilitation

One's sexual function after prostate cancer treatment will never be better than it was before—the best it can be is the way it was preceding treatment. In general, the better the erectile function before treatment, the better the function after treatment.

The best predictors of recovery of erectile function are age (younger better), pre-treatment function (better functional patients fare better) and in the case of prostatectomy, the extent of preservation of the neurovascular bundles (bilateral nerve sparing better than unilateral better than sacrificing both nerves). Additional factors are body mass index (the healthier the BMI the better), medical comorbidities (the fewer medical issues the better) and the skill and experience of the surgeon (more skilled and experienced better).

It is crucial to understand that "nerve-sparing" prostatectomy does not mean "immediate nerve-functioning," as it can take a considerable amount of time for nerve and erection recovery, even when the surgery is performed by the most skilled of robotic urological surgeons. Erectile function typically gradually improves over time, sometimes taking 2 years or more until optimal function returns.

After prostatectomy, there is most often a period of time in which the nerves to the erectile chambers remain in a state of dormancy, with decreased nitric oxide (the principal agent responsible for relaxation of penile smooth muscle) production and failure of nerve conduction resulting in the inability to obtain or maintain an erection and therefore the loss of the capacity for penetrative sexual intercourse. Recall that it is vital to obtain erections in order to maintain erections and that erections not only provide the capacity for penetrative sex, but also serve to prevent disuse atrophy by keeping the erectile smooth muscles and tissues richly oxygenated, elastic and functioning well. The consequence of the prolonged penile flaccidity that can occur after prostatectomy is scarring and damage to the erectile tissues. This often leads to venous leakage in which the penile blood trapping mechanism fails to work properly, further impeding rigidity and durability of erections—thus the importance of efforts directed at the expeditious resumption of erectile function, known as penile rehabilitation, to prevent the occurrence of this vicious cycle and optimize long-term erectile function.

Penile rehabilitation (Penile "rehab")

The purpose of penile rehab is to maintain penile blood flow during the time of nerve recovery so as to preserve and optimize future erectile function. Penile rehab makes use of specific exercises, medications and devices to enhance the recovery of erections and sexual function after prostate cancer treatment. Much like physical therapy used to rehabilitate injured body parts, penile rehabilitation is in essence the concept of physical therapy applied to the penis.

Instituting penile rehab as soon as feasible following prostatectomy helps provide a workable erection to enable sexual intercourse, maintain penile oxygenation and erectile tissue integrity, and hasten the resolution of sexual as well as urinary control issues. Those men who commit to a penile rehab program benefit from increased erection recovery rates and a better response to oral ED medications compared to those men who do not. Failure to participate in a penile rehab program may compromise and possibly jeopardize future erectile function.

The partner of the prostate cancer survivor can play a key role in his sexual recovery by providing emotional and psychological support, resulting in better adherence to the erection recovery program, improved sexual functioning and increased relationship satisfaction.

The starting point for penile rehab is usually the oral ED medications, which should be initiated as soon as possible after surgery to maintain erectile tissue oxygenation and prevent scarring. Many urologists prescribe daily low-dose Cialis or Viagra in the immediate post-operative period and continue this regimen for as long as necessary. An alternative is using higher doses of these or alternative ED medications two or three times weekly. The oral ED medications require functioning nerves to work properly, so even if they do not seem to help initially, they will start helping the situation as nerve recovery slowly occurs. Recent clinical trials have clearly demonstrated that early penile rehabilitation with oral ED medications immediately following catheter removal significantly improves erection recovery compared to delayed penile rehab starting several months after prostatectomy.

If the first-line oral ED medications do not result in sufficient erectile rigidity after a few weeks of trial, other penile rehab techniques can be used (while continuing the use of the ED medications, since erection recovery is an ongoing process).

Second-line rehab possibilities include penile injection therapy, vacuum erection devices and penile vibration therapy. In many cases it takes a combination of methods to optimize the return of erectile function. The best and most reliable alternatives for penile rehab are vacuum erection devices and vasodilator injections. The vacuum erection device is typically used for a total of 10 minutes daily, specifically 5 sets of 2-minute inflations, without using the tensioning ring. Alternatively, vasodilator injections are recommended to be used three times weekly. In either case, penile blood flow and erectile tissue integrity can be effectively maintained during the period of nerve recovery.

Pelvic floor muscle training, which ideally commenced prior to the prostatectomy, should be continued post-operatively since it contributes to recovery of both erections and urinary control.

Penile pre-rehab (Penile "prehab")

Prehab is a preemptive strategy that helps one prepare for the potential side effects of prostatectomy during the time interval between the establishment of the cancer diagnosis and the performance of the prostatectomy. This "proactive" as opposed to "reactive" approach can help prevent the occurrence of erectile and urinary control issues.

Once the diagnosis of prostate cancer is made, there are often several weeks prior to the scheduled surgery date. While this is obviously an emotionally fraught time, it can be put to beneficial use by having the patient physically prepare for the surgery to help prevent side effects. Aside from the physical benefits of prehab, it can also have a meaningful psychological and emotional impact. Prehab enables patients to take an active role in readying for surgery as well as facilitating recovery in the post-operative period, empowering them throughout the process.

Prehab includes pelvic floor muscle training and healthy lifestyle measures including a wholesome and nutritious diet, weight management, regular exercise and the cessation of tobacco usage. Pelvic floor muscle training increases the strength and endurance of the pelvic floor muscles that contribute to urinary control and erectile rigidity. Numerous clinical studies have demonstrated the benefits of pelvic floor muscle training *after* prostate surgery in decreasing the duration and severity of urinary control and sexual issues. Mastering pelvic floor muscle exercises *prior* to surgery confers the advantage of going into surgery with a fit and optimized pelvic floor, as well as learning the exercises under ideal circumstances that will result in the effortless resumption of the exercises in the post-operative period.

As the most expedient means of achieving pelvic strengthening, I highly recommend the following exercise program (disclaimer: I am co-creator of the program, which I felt was strongly needed as no adequate source for pre- and post-surgery male pelvic floor training exercises existed): PelvicRx (www.PelvicRx.com). It is a well-designed and easy to use, follow-along, interactive 4-week pelvic training program that offers strengthening and endurance pelvic floor exercises. It provides education, guidance, training and feedback to confirm the engagement of the proper muscles. It is structured so that repetitions, contraction intensity and contraction duration are gradually increased over the course of the program. This progression is the key to optimizing pelvic strength and endurance.

The reader is also referred to a book I wrote on the topic of male pelvic floor training: *MALE PELVIC FITNESS: Optimizing Sexual and Urinary Health*, published in 2014 (www.MalePelvicFitness.com).

Note: For a nice selection of erection recovery products, visit the Urology Health Store: www.UrologyHealthStore.com

Index

vibration device, 185, 203, 221

Additional Resources

American Cancer Society: www.cancer.org

Cancer Care: www.cancercare.org

Cancer.net: www.cancer.net

Help for Cancer Caregivers: www.helpforcancercaregivers.org

Male care: www.malecare.org

Men's Health Network: www.menshealthnetwork.org

National Cancer Institute: www.cancer.gov

Prostate Cancer Foundation: www.prostatecancerfoundation.org

Prostate Cancer Research and Education Foundation: www.pcref.org

Prostate Cancer Research Institute: www.prostate-cancer.org

Prostate Conditions Education Council: www.prostateconditions.org

Prostate Health Education Network: www.prostatehealthed.org

Urology Care Foundation: www.urologyhealth.org

Us TOO Prostate Cancer Education and Support Network: www.ustoo.org

Zero—The End of Prostate Cancer: www.zerocancer.org

About The Author

Andrew Siegel is an Alpha Omega Alpha honor graduate of Chicago Medical School. He completed surgery internship and residency at North Shore University Hospital and urology residency at University of Pennsylvania School of Medicine. He then pursued a fellowship in voiding dysfunction, incontinence, and pelvic reconstructive surgery at UCLA School of Medicine. He joined Bergen Urological Associates (now merged into New Jersey Urology—the largest urology practice in the United States) and the staff of Hackensack Meridian Health—Hackensack University Medical Center in 1988.

Dr. Siegel is dual board-certified in urology and female pelvic medicine/ reconstructive surgery and is an Assistant Clinical Professor of Surgery at the Rutgers-New Jersey Medical School where he is actively involved in the training of urology residents. He will continue his academic involvement with the newly established Hackensack Meridian School of Medicine at Seton Hall University. He is a Castle Connolly Top Doctor New York Metro area and Top Doctor New Jersey.

Dr. Siegel has authored chapters in urology textbooks and has published a multitude of articles in professional journals. He is passionate about wellness advocacy and is the author of four previous books: *FINDING YOUR OWN FOUNTAIN OF YOUTH: The Essential Guide to Maximizing Health, Wellness, Fitness and Longevity*; *PROMISCUOUS EATING— Understanding and Ending Our Self-Destructive Relationship with Food*; *MALE PELVIC FITNESS: Optimizing Sexual and Urinary Health*; and *THE KEGEL FIX: Recharging Female Pelvic, Sexual, and Urinary Health*.

He lives in the greater New York City area with his wife and English springer spaniel and is thrilled to spend time with his three grown children. He enjoys reading, writing, tennis, golf, cycling, fitness and living "clean" and healthy.

Also By Andrew L. Siegel, M.D.

THE KEGEL FIX: Recharging Female Pelvic, Sexual & Urinary Health

MALE PELVIC FITNESS: Optimizing Sexual and Urinary Health

PROMISCUOUS EATING: Understanding and Ending Our Self-Destructive Relationship With Food

FINDING YOUR OWN FOUNTAIN OF YOUTH: The Essential Guide to Maximizing Health, Fitness, Wellness & Longevity

To order copies of Dr. Siegel's other books: www.AndrewSiegelMD.com

Printed in Great
Britain
by Amazon

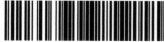